KIM'S STORY

A FIGHT FOR LIFE

KIM'S STORY

A FIGHT FOR LIFE

Scarlett McGwire

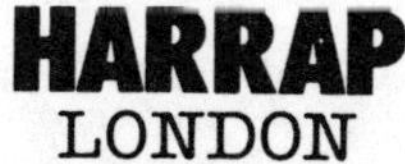

LONDON

First published in Great Britain 1986
by HARRAP Ltd
19-23 Ludgate Hill, London EC4M 7PD

ISBN 0 245-54396-1

Designed by Roger King Graphic Studios
Printed and bound in Great Britain
by Billing and Son, Worcester

To Duncan Campbell
who pulled us both through

CONTENTS

ILLUSTRATIONS

(Between pages 96 and 97)

ACKNOWLEDGMENTS

Kim's successful recovery was brought about with the help of our friends, family and the many nurses and doctors who cared for him. This book does not even begin to catalogue the kindness and support we received, neither does it portray the trauma suffered by Kim's family, in particular his parents. Every person mentioned did far more than I have written about, but in particular Mike Roberts and Jill Lourie did far more than the book gives them credit for. Many people are not mentioned at all. I would like to thank them all, particularly Angela Coles, Karen Douglas, John Hitchins, Vince McGarry and John Underwood.

The book was made possible with the encouragement and help of many people. John Gibbon, Richard Hayward and Barbara Wilson helped me with the information; Ursula Owen encouraged me to write it; Kate Holman pushed me when I almost gave up and Jane Gregory, Alison Peacock, Madeleine Colvin and Duncan Campbell all provided constructive criticism.

Susanna Klein looked after Pascoe while I wrote it.

I would like to thank all the people who appear in the book, but in particular my gratitude is to Kim who has allowed his personal tragedy to be made public in the hope that it will help someone else.

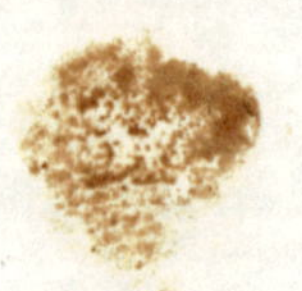

Chapter 1
THE ACCIDENT

Riding pillion behind Kim I looked over his shoulder and saw the bend coming. I knew we would not get round it. I cursed myself for not having made him slow down before, but it was too late now. The only chance of getting out of this lay with Kim. He needed total concentration. I forced myself to relax, to do nothing that would interfere, and prepared myself for the inevitable – feeling terribly vulnerable without the protection of a crash helmet. Life went into slow motion.

For a few brief moments it seemed we might escape. The bike rode up the red earth embankment which bordered the road, but it started bucking and I felt myself being thrown into the road.

Almost immediately I jumped up, glad to feel no bones broken, and surveyed the scene: the bike with its crumpled wheel, packages containing the presents we had been buying strewn across the road, and Kim lying, moaning, where he had been thrown. I swore loudly; then wondered how we were going to get back to our villa and what we were going to say to the man we had hired the bike from.

I felt a bit dizzy, put my hand to my head and felt something wet and sticky. It was blood. I sat down and gingerly probed all over my head, finding blood oozing back and front. I looked at my hands which were bleeding, saw blood all over my feet and more coming out of my knees. I was beginning to feel the wounds and bruises aching all over me.

Sitting on the tarmac on an empty Greek road, with not a person or house in sight, I started shouting pathetically for help.

A tourist bus coming along stopped and a coachload of Americans disembarked to help. The courier knew elementary first aid. She told us to lie still, putting towels under our heads to act as pillows and trying to calm us. The initial numbness caused by the shock was wearing off fast. I could feel every cut and bruise, which made me writhe in agony. I could hear Kim's loud moans and screams and saw that he too was flailing around as they unsuccessfully attempted to calm him and keep him still.

A pick-up truck appeared and we were loaded into it. To this day I have no idea how it came to be there; it was probably just passing. The Americans had packed up all our belongings and one of them gave me Kim's watch which had been scraped off his wrist in the fall. I clutched it like a rosary during the journey. A Greek man who spoke no English sat in the back with us.

As the truck started up I turned over to take Kim's hand and tell him everything would be all right now, we were on our way to hospital. But there was nothing. No response.

I shouted at the man in terror: "He's dead! He's dead!" Then I shouted at Kim that he must not die.

The man put his ear to Kim's chest and in sign language assured me that his heart was still beating. I could feel some relief.

Until we were in the truck it had not occurred to me that Kim could be significantly worse off than I was. My logic was simple: we had both come off the bike at roughly the same time; I was all right, therefore he would be. He had certainly been screaming more loudly as we lay by the road, but he had always made an enormous fuss about any injury so I had automatically allowed for that. I suppose the difference was that I had had nothing to hold on to so came off easily and landed lightly because I was relaxed, whereas Kim would have been grappling with the handlebars until the last minute when he was catapulted off much more forcefully.

I was on the Greek island of Rhodes, spoke barely a word of the language, with my boyfriend possibly dying beside me and both of us at the mercy of strangers. It was the beginning of a nightmare that was to take so many twists and turns I wondered at times if it would ever end.

I lay back in the truck and remembered our life as it had been only minutes ago – when we appeared to have an eternity together.

I remembered the first time I set eyes on Kim – less than two years earlier. I was a reporter for Independent Radio News, the news service for all commercial ratio stations. There had been a lot of talk about Kim Sabido joining us from BRMB, the Birmingham radio station; the news editor had been trying to tempt him down for weeks while Kim had procrastinated. I was interested to see the man who had caused all the fuss.

When he walked through the door, academic curiosity changed to admiration – nobody had mentioned that as well as being an excellent reporter he was very good-looking – classically tall, dark and handsome.

I was having an enjoyable affair which I knew had no future, so I made a mental note to take some action when I was free.

In the ensuing months Kim developed into a fascinating enigma for me. I found him temptingly unapproachable which I put down to arrogance. Judging by the stories other reporters had recounted of their sexual exploits when they were in the regions I assumed he had had his pick of women in Birmingham and had no interest in me.

By this time I was working on the weekend programmes for LBC, the London news station that works out of the same office as IRN. One Saturday evening Kim did an interview for the programme and informed me I would have to do all the work to get it ready to go to air because his shift had finished and he had a pressing engagement to go to. This was not common practice, and I was not pleased. When I had finished the work, Kim was still messing around in the office – so much for the pressing engagement. The next morning I gave him hell, telling him he was an arrogant swine and in future he could do his own dirty work, I was not there to clean up after him.

He was quite clearly mortified. My sharp words had so successfully deflated him that I was nice to him for the rest of the day to show I was not really angry, just making a point. We went for a drink afterwards, then for a Chinese meal, and I told a series of stories against myself to try and make him laugh at me. It was an extremely pleasant evening and I came away with a vital bit of information: there was no girlfriend.

It was almost December and the usual round of parties meant it took me a while to follow up the initial breakthrough. Then just before Christmas the Penlee lifeboat sank going to the aid of a stricken ship, and Kim was sent to Cornwall. He did not reappear until mid-January. When he returned I decided that any procrastination could mean another long wait until Kim returned from another story, so we saw each other the next Saturday night, and romance blossomed.

It was a pleasant surprise to learn Kim was not the suave confident man he appeared but one of the shyest people I have ever met in journalism. It had not been a case of being too disdainful to hold a conversation with me, but my reputation as a sharp-tongued feminist, which I found a convenient shield to protect my own vulnerability, had made him so terrified of saying the wrong thing he preferred to keep quiet.

His grandfather had come to Britain from Belize in Central America to fight in the First World War, and settled in Wales. Kim's father married a young Welsh girl and moved with her to Bristol to find work. They had four children: Richard, Roger, Sue and the youngest Kim. Mr Sabido was a strong patriarchal figure who wanted the best for his children. He ensured they were all brought up in the Catholic faith and the boys sent to a Christian Brothers school. He was extremely disappointed when Kim, unlike his elder siblings, chose not to go to university; instead he wanted to be a journalist. Kim's Aunt Mala got him his first job at the *Merthyr Express*, and for the next few years he worked on papers in South Wales, teaching himself Welsh and rediscovering his Welsh roots – his mother had not learned English until she was thirteen.

On the *Glamorgan Gazette* in Bridgend Kim met a fellow reporter, Pat Hurley, who had returned to journalism after bringing up her four sons. She took him in as her lodger, and he became part of the family. After a spell as a freelance he landed his first radio job on Radio Forth in Edinburgh.

His stories of Radio Forth made it sound like a madhouse, which will come as no surprise to anybody who has come into close contact with any Independent Radio station. With no radio experience at all he was hired as Sports Editor and was promised a trip to Argentina for the 1978 World Cup if Scotland qualified. He did the commentary for all of Scotland's qualifying games, including the notorious match against Wales, in which all but the most ardent Scots supporters agree that the referee missed an important foul which cost Wales the game. Not only did Kim have to watch the terrible defeat, he had to commentate from the Scots point of view. Then someone else was sent to Argentina – Kim had lost out in the office politicking. He was furious.

After a few months as a general reporter he returned to Wales to work on Swansea Sound. There he lived with Ian Parkinson who is now on *Newsbeat*, and a young trainee David Johnstone who went on to Radio Forth where he is now the news editor.

The next move was to BRMB in Birmingham where Kim shared a house with Andrew Burn, a solicitor and fellow sports fanatic. Andrew's partners in his firm of solicitors were Colin Viner and Peter Millichip, and the three were Kim's closest friends in Birmingham. Peter's father was Bert Millichip who was chair of West Bromwich Albion and is now chair of the Football Association, so West Brom became Kim's second favourite football team, after Cardiff City naturally.

Kim was very happy in Birmingham, which was why he was so reluctant to go to London to join IRN. When he finally took the job, Andrew was certain he would return to the city within months, if not to BRMB then to a job with Central Television there.

Andrew was not far wrong. Kim hated London. He enjoyed his work but outside the office he was desperately lonely, and returned to Birmingham most weekends. Circumstances there had changed, however, because Andrew's new girlfriend found Kim's presence intrusive. I happened along at just the right moment.

Kim told me he had chosen journalism as the only job that would get him over his terrible shyness and everybody had laughed when he had first voiced his ambition. I had chosen journalism because it seemed the only job that would provide enough variety to keep me from getting bored. My life had been built on perpetual change. My father was in the Royal Navy. By the time I was eleven I was about to start on my seventh school, had lived in the Soviet Union and America (with a sister born in the former and a brother in the latter), and all over the south of England.

A significant proportion of my life had also been spent in hospital. When I was eleven weeks old I was given two hours to live because of a defective kidney. My life was saved by an operation to remove it, but by this time the remaining kidney was also damaged. When my parents finally took me home, my mother was warned that I would not make eighteen months – a cheering thing to be told about your first child.

The next eight years were spent waiting for medicine to catch up with the problem before the kidney gave out, for those were the days before transplants, which meant months in hospital.

I was lucky. In America a surgeon came up with an operation that fixed the kidney and apart from a distinct lack of physical stamina I am now remarkably healthy. I have lived through enough scare diagnoses always to listen with a degree of scepticism to any doctor.

I had two more schools to go through after I was eleven, a Dorset comprehensive with boarding facilities, which I found extraordinarily oppressive, and Atlantic College which is an international sixth form college, now part of a network of schools, which I found great fun because it was so easy to run riot. Apparently it has since changed and is much more serious. I went to Canada for a year after that, where I got a job as a journalist, and found it difficult to come back to go to university which seemed like an extended school after the 'real world'; I learned little about my degree subject, psychology, and a fair amount about Marxism.

I went on the Mirror Group Newspapers training scheme in Plymouth and left after eighteen months, mostly to escape from a dreadful man with whom I was having a disastrous relationship. In London I freelanced in Fleet Street for a while, got a six-month contract with the BBC World Service, then joined IRN where I stayed for almost four years doing various jobs. I also became active in the National Union of Journalists, and many of my friends came from there.

Kim shared my politics, although being a man he did not have to fight on all fronts at once, trying to do something about the position of women as well as everything else.

I was extremely tentative with Kim at first, quite happy with a relaxed casual relationship, kept firmly under wraps at work. But over a couple of months it became more serious. At the end of March I went to the NUJ annual delegate meeting at Warwick University for five days. I returned on the Friday night and raced off to Cardiff to speak at a conference. On the Sunday Kim had to go into work and after six days of late nights, heavy debates and too much drink I could finally have a restful day.

That afternoon I was slowly getting myself unpacked and organized when Kim suddenly burst in on me and said we had to go to Portsmouth immediately. A task force was being sent to the Falklands and IRN had chosen him to go on it. It was all too unreal for me to get worked up about, and when we arrived there we discovered there had been a mistake. He did not have a place on either *Hermes* or *Invincible*, but a troop carrier was following and he would be on that.

There was still the possibility of everything being called off but as I watched the task force leave Portsmouth the next morning to the cheers of the crowds on the docks I felt quite sick. The patriotic fervour and jingoism was unnerving, particularly as most of the people on the quayside had only the vaguest idea of where the Falklands were. Watching those crews standing to attention on deck, I wondered how many would return.

Five days later Kim was on the *Canberra* with the marines, a parachute regiment and a motley bunch of journalists, slowly wending his way to the South Atlantic. And I was left to wonder about his fate.

It was to be three months before I saw him again. In that time he learned at first hand that war was not about bravery and heroism but about being scared and uncomfortable. The reports he sent back were labelled left wing, but in fact he was just giving the point of view of the soldiers rather than keeping up the morale of those back home. He spoke scathingly of the claret-swilling politicians; he felt the soldiers had to risk their lives because of the mistakes of the politicians.

He spent a terrifying two hours on an ammunition ship during an Argentinian bombing raid – one direct hit and the ship would have been blown to kingdom come, taking most of the harbour with it. He was the only journalist to go into the front line for the last battle in the war, when he watched an officer who had befriended him, Ian Stafford, shot in the knee beside him. He swore he would never meaninglessly risk his life again.

Those three months were extremely odd for me; from the day he landed on the islands until the war was over I had no contact with him, I only knew he was alive when he was on the radio. My friends said I was lucky because at least I had that, but for the forces' wives and girlfriends there was the comradeship of all being the same boat, they could support each other, while I knew no one who had a physical stake in the war. I opposed it on moral and political grounds; above all I could not comprehend how people could go and kill other people on the orders of a government.

When Kim returned it was ecstasy. We were just blissfully happy.

Before he went away he had been offered a job by Independent Television News as a reporter and after a holiday with me in Spain he went to work for them. Joining ITN was achieving the peak of his ambition, something he had never really thought possible.

I had been trying to leave LBC for over a year, but one scheme after another fell through. Finally just before Christmas I resigned, with nothing particular to go to. A friend of mine, Anna Coote, whom I had met at my first union annual delegate meeting in 1980, was working for a Channel Four company, Diverse Productions, who were producing *The Friday Alternative* and she persuaded me to do some work for them. A few days turned into weeks which turned into months. The hours and demands were appalling but I enjoyed it immensely.

Kim and I decided to buy a house and live together because the pressures of our work meant that, living in our separate flats, we hardly ever saw each other.

Life was wonderful, we were both doing fulfilling work, on good salaries, still in love; the only real disagreement was that I wanted to get pregnant immediately and Kim wanted to wait a year or two. He liked our freewheeling lifestyle, which would be constricted by a child.

I vividly remember standing in his kitchen in February 1983 thinking of our lives and how our only problem was the prospect at boredom with the blissful future mapped out in front of us. Everything seemed just too perfect.

When I discovered I was pregnant in March it was as if we had been favoured by the gods – I was so happy. Even Kim found the imminent prospect of fatherhood exciting. It caused a few problems at Diverse, partly because of the complete lack of sympathy with the effects of my condition, which were continuous nausea and mind-numbing tiredness, partly because I had just begun to negotiate a contract of employment. Eventually I was given a contract that would take me up to my proposed maternity leave, which gave me a bit of security.

We moved into the new house the day before the pregnancy was confirmed, a ramshackle Victorian heap in urgent need of repairs and decoration, bought purely on the grounds of its enormous potential. From the time of our move we hardly seemed to see each other, with me working during the week and Kim sent to Belfast at the weekends. When he was sent there for Easter, in spite of us having booked a holiday in Wales and hired a farmhouse to stay in, I felt so depressed I decided to follow him out there. He was put on a wild goose chase looking for the missing racehorse Shergar, and I did not see much of him as he made two trips to Dublin that weekend. To pay for my fare I found a story I could do there for Diverse and went to Derry to interview the relations of a man who had been kidnapped by the INLA. When I returned to London Kim had important news for me – he was being sent to the Falklands for three months. ITN wanted him to cover the first anniversary of the war.

I cursed ITN. I was about ten weeks pregnant and during a time that I needed support badly Kim was not just going to be physically separated from me but communications were going to be difficult as phone calls out of the islands were heavily rationed.

I was at a union conference in Dundee when he left five days later and the next week worked hard enough to keep myself from missing him. By the time I went to my first antenatal appointment three weeks after he had left I was feeling terrible with the pregnancy but able to cope with his absence. Then the doctor told me I had probably had a miscarriage because my womb was not the size it should be and no heartbeat could be found on the scan. The technical term was a missed abortion because I still had the foetus in my womb. I went home that night so I could have a conversation with Kim, which was dreadful. He had been unable to phone out so ITN had rung him, then rung me and put the phones together so we could talk to each other. It was no intimate conversation but shouted terse sentences. The ITN Foreign Editor Maggie Eales had told Kim the problem. He asked what was the matter with the baby. I answered that it was probably a chromosome defect, as I did not want to tell him it could have been overwork. Kim misheard me and as he was flown home that night to be me, he kept asking the people on the plane what a cortisone baby was, thinking it was so terrible I would never be able to have children.

I had a D & C to remove the foetus from my womb the next day and soon after I woke up from the operation Kim was at my bedside.

That was twelve days ago – this holiday had been for me to recuperate from the operation and for both of us to get over the miscarriage, and it all seemed to have gone terribly wrong.

As we were driven along in the battered truck, Kim's breathing turned into a rasping effort. Was this a death rattle? The Greek also heard but he looked at me with a gesture of helplessness: neither of us could do anything.

In a small town, off the main road, we pulled up at what I assumed was a doctor's surgery from the medical cross outside it. Faces crowded over the sides of the truck to peer at us. A man fought his way through to us, looked at Kim, shook his head at the man in the truck, said a few words and we drove off. Somehow I was made to understand that he was a doctor who felt the case was too serious for his limited local facilities, and we were going on to the hospital in Rhodes Town.

Lying prone in the back of the truck, shaken by every bump in the badly made up road, a towel acting as a pillow to cushion my head, I watched the sun slowly set and felt the temperature begin to drop during the seemingly interminable journey, though I knew from the distance involved it could not have taken more than an hour. I alternated between dread that Kim would not be alive at the end and envy at his unconscious state: this was a memory I had no wish to retain.

When we finally arrived at the hospital the truck was once again surrounded by people; I was discovering the attraction a drama holds for the Greeks.

They carried Kim out on a stretcher first. As I waited, a man, an American I think, leaned over and told me God would look after us both, all I had to do was trust in God and it would be all right. To an aetheist like me those were hardly words of comfort; my immediate response was guilt and the feeling that I would be responsible for Kim's death because I had no faith. Over the next twenty-four hours I behaved not as an unbeliever, but as someone who had had a serious rift with God: I lay staring at the ceiling and cursed what He had done to Kim or implored Him to look after His own because Kim was still a believer. He was not to take my failings out on an innocent boy. At least it gave me someone to shout at apart from myself. I was wracked with guilt: I had suggested hiring the bike and when Kim had said it was too hot to wear a crash helmet I had not argued.

In casualty they examined Kim, put a catheter on his bladder, stuck a drip in his arm and wheeled him off for an x-ray. The doctor, who had been trained in London so spoke English, told me Kim was seriously ill and he was not sure he would recover. He said those stark words with such concern that I felt he would do everything possible to save him.

By this time I was in a state of such physical and mental shock that I could barely speak. The hospital needed to know all sorts of details, but it was a great effort getting command of my vocal chords to say my name, it took all the concentration I could muster to spell it out, spell Kim's, tell them where we were staying, which tour operator we were with and remember the name of our courier. Luckily a German nurse spoke English and was wonderfully reassuring as she patiently allowed me to stutter out the information.

They decided I needed a shot of Largactyl to calm me down. I knew, from having cut my head open before, that people with head injuries, however minor, should not be given any sort of sedative, because if they become unconscious it is difficult to know whether it is delayed concussion or due to the medication. I had also heard enough dreadful things about Largactyl, used to calm rioting prisoners and mental patients and known as the liquid cosh, not to want it under any circumstances; but the thought of trying to get through the language barrier, overcome my physical state and thwart the will of the doctors almost brought on tears of helplessness, so I just let them inject it.

After examining me the doctor told me I had no serious injuries. On the one hand I felt relief but also frustration that they could dismiss my pains so easily. I had two bad gashes on my head, one on my forehead and the other at the back and my hands were badly cut from trying to break my fall. Luckily I had put on a jump suit for the journey or the grazing would have been far more serious for I could feel bruises developing all over me from where I had been thrown from the bike and slid along the tarmac. My knees and ankles were swelling and I found it difficult to walk without help for days, it was to be weeks before the swellings went down.

While the nurse did her best to alleviate my suffering, gently bathing my wounds and putting a few stitches in my head, trying all the while not to hurt me, another examining doctor, unfortunately not the same man as Kim's, inflicted as much unnecessary pain as possible, even to the extent of testing my reflexes five times by tickling the soles of my feet when he realised I hated it. The next afternoon he asked me how I was and when I shrugged and said that compared to Kim I was all right but I was feeling pretty awful, he just slapped my oozing open head wound and said there was nothing wrong with me, leaving me stunned and hurting.

After casualty had patched me up I was sent to be x-rayed, where they cut my clothes off me and replaced them with regulation pyjamas, which I still have as a memento of my stay. The two technicians smoked constantly as they worked the machine. This shocked me terribly but I was soon to learn that this hospital was not run on the strict codes of hygiene and discipline prevalent in English ones.

After I had been wheeled through my ward, with a porter kindly pointing out Kim's room on the way, I realised I had to go to the loo. The nurse was remarkably quick at understanding my need for a bed-pan, in spite of speaking no English, but bemused when I pulled the bedclothes up to try and give me some privacy – there were no curtains.

As the Largactyl took effect I slipped into a semi-conscious stupor with periods of drifting off perpetually interrupted by people asking me questions and trying to get answers out of me. My ward was the throughway to the lavatory, and every woman going that way made a detour to my bed to make a close inspection of me. I seemed to be a star attraction. The other women in the room with me had to give all my details to the other curious patients, who would then kindly pat me on the head and utter some reassuring sounding words. A hospital administrator came to get all my details and find out about our medical insurance, to ensure the hospital was going to be paid.

Then the visit I had been dreading – the police. Kim had not been insured for driving the bike, only me, because his licence was in England being endorsed for a speeding offence. I did not want any wrangles with the Greek authorities about insurance so I told the police the whole story, correct in every detail that I could remember, except I claimed I had been driving. Natural chauvinism must have made them wonder why a woman was driving but they did not appear to doubt the story. I did not realise that in most accidents the pillion passenger comes off worse, which supported my story. They were not interested in making a fuss. They were quite content for me to admit that thirty miles an hour was rather fast considering my inexperience and leave it at that. As far as they were concerned, two foreigners had injured themselves in an accident caused by them and involving no one else. End of story. Case closed. Any charges seemed irrelevant.

My next awakening was to the British Vice-Consul. By this time it was nearing midnight. He went through the details from our passports, the tour company we were with, our courier and the medical insurance. Then he wanted to know the names of our next of kin. I said I did not want any dramatic middle-of-the-night phone calls which would worry people unnecessarily; when it was all over people could be told.

There was a slight pause. Then he told me that what I decided to do about my next of kin was up to me, because my injuries were only superficial; but for Kim it was different. The doctors had diagnosed a fractured skull and he was in a critical condition. His life was in danger, so his next of kin must be informed.

I remembered when Kim had gone to cover the Falklands war he had given his brother-in-law, Paul Steele, as next of kin because he felt that if the worst were to happen Paul would be the most appropriate person to receive the news and disseminate it around the family. So I gave Paul's name and address and explained that I did not have his phone number, but to note that as he had only just moved to Winchester it could be found under new numbers through Directory Enquiries.

There were no appropriate facilities for Kim on the island; the only chance for him was to be flown home and treated there. I gave the Vice-Consul all the practical information which would be useful in getting a plane over as fast as possible. We had holiday medical insurance that gave twenty-four-hour air ambulance cover, so I did not envisage any problems. I remembered reading all the details the night before we flew. The documents were in our villa in Lindos; I did not know its address but if he contacted the Timsway courier there, Jill, she would be able to pick them up and get all the relevant details so the plane could be sent. He went away to phone Jill.

When the Vice-Consul left I had a chance to consider the news he had given me. My first reaction was one of relief: finally I knew what was wrong. With my limited medical knowledge I did not regard a fractured skull as some terrible injury, just a bad bang on the head. As a journalist I only knew about fractured skulls from stories I had covered, and the people always seemed to get better. (Of course stories picked up by the media are by their very nature always the exception, never the rule.) I felt quite optimistic about Kim's chances. It was now just a matter of getting him home so he could have proper medical attention; I had no idea of the yawning gap between what was needed and what he was getting.

I knew three cheering examples of serious head injuries. The girlfriend of Paul Davies, whom I had worked with at IRN and is now an ITN reporter, had been in a car crash and for weeks afterwards had been in a coma. At first she had not been expected to live, and if she did come round it was assumed she would be mentally and physically handicapped for the rest of her life. When I met her a year or so later she appeared perfectly normal and was back at her job as a PE teacher.

Alvin was an engineer at LBC/IRN. He had been nearly murdered by a man bashing in his skull in while he was in the bath. There were fears for his life, but ten days later he had come out of his coma and within a year was back at work, with little change apart from losing his peripheral vision.

Finally, there was Stephen Waldorf, the man shot then pistol whipped by the police in a case of mistaken identity. Kim had covered the story for ITN from the day Stephen was shot until he was finally let out of hospital. We had talked of little else throughout that time. I remembered the days when Stephen's life hung in the balance and also recalled assuming that first evening that it would be better if he did not live because he would be a vegetable afterwards. The interview Kim did with Stephen a few weeks later showed him as lucid as anybody. Stephen was a tiny frail man, whereas Kim was a great strapping fellow. I was sure he could do as well, and unlike Stephen he did not have bullets in his brain.

Yes, everything would be all right once the plane arrived and we could get Kim back to England. Those three success stories were to pull me through the next few days: every time I felt despondent about Kim's recovery I would repeat those facts and cheer myself up.

It was another part of the Vice-Consul's visit that worried me far more. When he asked how the accident had happened, so the basic details could be communicated to Kim's family, I had explained about the story I had had to tell the police because of the insurance problems, but asked if he could ensure the correct story was transmitted to England. He refused and said the official version would have to be communicated; no amount of pleading would change his mind. How was I going to face Kim's parents? They did not approve of me at the best of times, but now they were to be told I was responsible for almost killing their son. They would assume that my feminist notions had led me to insist on driving. If Kim did not recover, he would be able to support my story and I would probably never be believed.

There was no sleep for me that night, partly because of worry over that and the worse thought of poor Kim's family being woken up by the news, then just having to sit out the night waiting to hear of his fate; but mainly because of the after-effects of the Largactyl. It had been given with an intermuscular injection and my arm was a terrible constant ache – any pleasant effects of the drug had long since worn off. The nurse brought me sleeping-pills, but they had no effect, and I was left listening to the night sounds of the hospital, at one stage pierced by a child crying for his mother, followed by a stretcher being wheeled past my door. I gathered later that she too had been in a motorbike accident but had not survived.

I was desperate to get to sleep so that the night would pass quickly and I could wake up, get on the plane, and all the awfulness would be over.

While I was lying awake, feeling my head wounds still oozing, I had the alarming thought that I might be more damaged than anyone had noticed and could be suffering from brain damage. I decided to test out the various parts of my brain to check they were all in working order. To do this I set myself difficult mental arithmetic problems and concentrated on different areas of my brain to do them. So the front bit multiplied 193 by 98, then the back part divided 3679 by 23, and I made the sides and middle bits do various other problems. By the end I was satisfied I had a whole brain in working order. I later realised that if there was a sign that I was completely round the bend it was doing that test at all, believing I could choose which parts of my brain I put to work; but it kept me happy and occupied, and my insanity was harmless.

At about six the next morning Jill the courier came to see me. She had spent the night at the hospital but had not been allowed to see me before because the nurse did not want my sleep disturbed. As she had had to give me sleeping-pills after Jill's arrival I could not follow the logic, but let it pass. Jill had spent the night fitfully dozing on a bench outside Kim's room, because no one else appeared to be paying him any attention at all. His breathing was still rasping and uneven, and many times during the night she had woken in a panic to hear nothing and gone in to check on him, thinking he had died. She reported he was still alive, though unconscious and receiving scant medical attention. It was only later we realised that he had just been left to die because there were no medical facilities to deal with his condition.

On Jill's arrival I had expected Kim and me to begin our trip to the airport so we could board the plane and go home, but I discovered there was no waiting plane. Jill had rung our medical insurance company, Medex, as soon as she had heard about the accident to request an emergency air ambulance, but the person on duty had said she would have to wait until morning when the company doctor could speak to the Greek doctors. We now had to wait until 9 a.m. British time, which was two hours behind Greek time, to telephone again. I was bitterly disappointed to discover that far from being about to be rescued, the operation was still in the planning stages. I remembered the terms of the insurance which gave not only twenty-four-hour cover but implied that planes would fly to any part of the world at the summons of a phone call.

In spite of my optimism about Kim I felt he needed help fast if he was to recover.

I tried to be quite cheery when I spoke to Jill, partly because it was so good to speak to someone who understood English and who appreciated the problems and was going to sort them out, partly because I was trying to view the whole episode as an adventure which, however unpleasant it might be just now, would be amusing to recount when I got home. As Jill left to buy some anti-tetanus drugs for us (the hospital did not run to such medication) and unravel more administrative red tape I tried to look positively at the situation. I felt I was experiencing a part of Greece that as a tourist soaking up the sun on beaches I could never have reached. I was still the centre of much attention in my room, as every woman paying her morning visit to the loo would come over and offer a few words of comfort. For years I had wanted to make a film about the enigma of Greek women, most of whom seemed inaccessible to the tourist, now here I was surrounded by them.

Suddenly, as I was trying to jolly myself along and keep up my spirits, I just snapped and burst into tears. Here I was, lying in a foreign hospital bed aching all over from my wounds, unable to walk or even sit up for more than a few minutes without lapsing into spells of dizziness, with my head injuries still oozing and flies all over the place, which had probably given me some dreadful disease; if that was not enough, my boyfriend was critically ill, maybe dying, along the corridor, with nobody doing anything about it, and it was going to be hours before there was any hope of being taken away from it all.

I immersed myself in self-pity having decided I was sick of keeping the famous British stiff upper lip and always looking for the positive side of any disaster that hit me. I had even managed to see my miscarriage as showing that I was not sterile, so at least would be able to conceive again. Now it looked as though I might lose the boyfriend as well as the baby. There was a fresh surge of tears at the thought.

The sympathetic Greek women tried to cheer me up and stop the weeping, but I just wanted to be left alone to go on crying.

Eventually I managed to distract my mind by turning it to the more practical problem of how to avoid being given a bed-bath by a rough nurse. I was covered in dried blood and dreaded the pain of having the scabs pulled off. A long soak in a bath would be the best way to clean me and get the worst of the blood off; it might also do a little to ease all the aches. When the nurse next came into the room I attempted to explain my request. She and one of the patients supported my journey to the bathroom and took me into the shower, a primitive type with nothing more than a faucet and a cracked base. I made it clear that I could not have a shower because I could not stand up. I had to have a bath. So they took me to the basin. Again I explained that the problem was that I could not stand. It had to be a bath. They took me back to my bed and slowly I began to understand that there were no baths. I had just been given a tour of the available washing facilities.

I need not have worried about the roughness of a bed-bath: Rhodian nursing did not extend to such luxuries. In that hospital if anyone needed washing, relatives or friends came in to do it, otherwise the patient stayed dirty. I managed to get some of the caked blood off by being innovative with the contents of my lunch tray and dipping the paper napkin into the glass of water; that got the worst off my forearms but I could not even begin on my face because there was no mirror.

During the morning I received regular bulletins from Jill on her fruitless attempts to get Medex moving with an air ambulance. No plane would be sent until someone had spoken to a hospital doctor, but nobody from Medex could get through to the hospital switchboard and the hospital refused to let the doctors make any calls to Britain because of the cost. It was not a matter of crossing a palm with silver; we tried everything. We were stuck trying to get two immovable objects to meet. Jill was pleading with both sides, but neither was budging an inch.

I was equally unsuccessful in persuading anyone to let me see Kim. I was unable to take matters into my own hands because I could not walk and anyway could not locate his whereabouts from the vague memory of the night before when his room was pointed out to me. I could not enlist Jill's help against the doctors because she was trying desperately to persuade them to do something to get the plane in the air. She had seen him and had discussed his condition with the doctors: he was in a bad way and deteriorating. I was left lying in my bed with the constant dread that every nurse, doctor or hospital official walking into the room had come to tell me Kim had died. Finally after lunch someone relented. There were no wheelchairs available so I was put in a commode and wheeled down to Kim's room.

He was unconscious but breathing. In my medical ignorance I thought he looked remarkably well, his beautifully tanned, lithe body was rising and falling as he took regular, deep breaths. Surely nobody looking that brown and healthy could be near death?

With tears running down my face I took his hand and started talking, not to try and bring him round, I thought he was probably better off not knowing about all this, but to reassure him that he was not alone and encourage him to go on fighting to stay alive. I told him to hang on a bit longer because we were getting a plane to fly him to England, which should arrive in a few hours; then everything would be all right because he would be looked after properly and would be able to relax and let other people do the work. To persuade him to fight to stay alive I told him all the things that the thought of him dying had made me realise: just how much I needed him and how much better a person he had made me because I no longer felt I had to take on the world single-handed; if he did not stay around I would return to being an embittered old battleaxe. And I apologised for all the times I had been appalling to him.

I am sure I made many promises about how things would change if only he would get better, and I must have broken every one since. The one I remember and the one I just about kept for a few months was swearing to put him first in my life until he got better. In the past it had not been just a matter of putting myself first, he had also come a bad second to my job, my union activities and any other matters of political conscience. The job's priority he accepted and ITN expected the same from him, but when I spent time during our few days off together in union meetings or negotiations his patience was tried.

As I watched his chest steadily rise and fall I thought of his father who suffered from the wasting lung disease emphysema and was virtually written off about three years earlier after a very bad attack. He had survived and was still alive because of a strong heart and sheer bloody willpower. I knew Kim had inherited the cussedness and I just prayed he had the heart as well.

Kim was in a normal public ward like mine, and while I had been prevented from visiting him, presumably because they were worried I might become hysterical, anybody else could take a look, and did. Every patient in the corridor appeared to know about us and they and their visitors would come and gawp. Unlike British hospitals, there were neither set visiting hours nor the rather reverential tones used around sick people. Being in this hospital was like being in the middle of a rolling cocktail party from early morning until well into the night; people turned up in crowds with food and drink and chattered away at the tops of their voices. None of the other patients appeared to be upset by the lack of peace and quiet.

After I had sat beside Kim's bed for about an hour they decided to move him to a single room. The reasoning was never explained. As his condition had stabilised since my being allowed to see him it was unlikely they feared his imminent demise and it was certainly not due to complaints from me; after my morning discovery of no baths I was quite prepared to believe the hospital did not stretch to separate rooms for the critically ill.

Perhaps it was a sign of optimism: his condition was now worth treating. For the first time since we had arrived at the hospital I witnessed some modern technology, not that it was put to particularly constructive use. They first produced a spray which when applied to oozing wounds acted as instant skin, sealing them. Both of us had this applied to our foreheads. Unfortunately it did not occur to anybody to wash the wounds first. The second new toy was an EEG machine to monitor the heart. It was obviously a recent acquisition because no one was quite sure how to use it. With the aid of the instruction booklet and by trial and error they fitted the suckers to Kim's chest and connected them to the machine so that the readings were satisfactory. Then they left the room. I could not understand why they had gone to the trouble of fitting up the machine. Nobody came to keep an eye on what was happening and there was no print-out, so it was not a matter of charting his progress over a period of time. The machine was facing away from me so that even my extremely limited knowledge, culled from television drama, could not be put to interpreting the patterns on the screen because I could not see them.

The move to a private room coupled with the exciting machine made us even more of a focal point for the curious. I sat there with a constant flow of tears running silently down my face, holding the hand of this comatose man lying still on the bed, trying to think of words which would bolster his spirits and keep him fighting, waiting for Jill to return with good news about the plane. I felt certain Kim could not survive another night without help. All the while patients and visitors came into the room in twos and threes to stare at us, nudge each other as they pointed at us and then start examining the EEG machine. Finally a nurse noticed what was going on and shooed a group out, then put a notice up on the door forbidding visitors.

Jill arrived with the first hint of good news about the plane: ITN had rung her office in Rhodes and left a message saying they were trying to get a plane for us. It was like hearing the bugles of the cavalry. I knew ITN would fix it and everything was going to be all right.

Jill and I pondered over how ITN had discovered our predicament. Much later I learned it was through my ineptitude over giving Kim's next of kin. Nobody had been able to locate his brother-in-law, but some bright spark at the Foreign Office had recognised Kim's name and had phoned ITN to begin the hunt for relatives. ITN treated the matter like a story, assigning people to the job of both locating Kim's next of kin and finding out what had happened. Not only did they manage to find one of Kim's brothers, they also got through to the hospital, discovered Kim's condition, learned about the trouble we were having getting an air ambulance and made sure Medex realised some rather influential people were quite concerned about Kim's fate and would be asking questions if something was not done about it pretty damn quick.

Within an hour of ITN's message Jill received a telex from Medex saying a plane was on its way from Manchester. We just clung to each other and cried.

Chapter 2
THE JOURNEY HOME

After the first rush of euphoria it became a matter of just settling down to more waiting. I longed for the plane to land so I could hand over responsibility for Kim to someone who knew how to look after him. I craved to be able to stop fighting for him, so I could sink into the oblivion I could feel overtaking me. I just wanted to wake up and find myself in England, to have someone looking after me and to know Kim was going to be all right.

All this would be possible when the plane arrived, but until then Kim was my responsibility. I squeezed his hand and told him the air ambulance was on its way; help would be here soon. I begged him to hang on a few more hours, he just had to keep fighting a little longer.

My throbbing head told me even sitting up was too much effort. I was growing dizzy. Jill helped me into the empty bed in the room so I could both rest and keep watch over Kim. She then returned to our villa to pack up our belongings ready for the flight. I lay on the bed trying to relax, attempting to speed the passing minutes.

As I lay there I wondered what would have happened to Kim if he had been Greek. If we had been rich we would have paid for a plane to take him to a good hospital in Athens, but failing that I would just have had to wait for him to die. The Greek government apportioned a tiny fraction of their GNP to health.

The imminent arrival of the air ambulance did not signal the end of our problems. First there was the question of the hospital bill. The rules stated that no patient could leave the hospital until the bill had been settled. Medex had no representative on the island to pay the cash so asked the hospital to invoice them. The hospital reiterated its position: no money, no discharge. Jill pointed out that Kim's life depended on reaching London, but the administrator just shrugged and said we should come up with the money. Only a pittance was involved so I knew it was merely a matter of muscles being flexed to prove a point, and someone would give way so Kim could leave, but it was unpleasant to be in the middle of the fight as it continued. Jill's colleagues from Timsway refused on principle to let me pay the money; we were insured for this eventuality and Medex should honour their commitment. As it was, Timsway had had to put their office resources into getting the air ambulance, which should have involved just one telephone call. In the end Timsway paid the bill through reluctant necessity.

When Jill returned with the luggage we were faced with another bureaucratic tangle. Before Kim would be allowed on the plane a Greek doctor had to sign a form saying the flight was medically necessary; but the doctors said the only man with that authority had gone on holiday for two weeks. None of the others were prepared to take the responsibility.

Neither reason nor pleading would move the doctors. When the Vice-Consul arrived to deliver some of our personal effects which had been given to him after the crash we explained the problem. He spoke to the doctors who immediately concurred with him that there must have been some misunderstanding and treated Jill and me as hysterical women concocting crises. Unfortunately all this man-to-man talk had only a temporary effect – as soon as the Vice-Consul left the doctors once again told us they would sign nothing. We were still having the argument when we heard Kim's plane overhead flying into the airport and about twenty minutes later saw the sweep of headlights through the window as the ambulance drew up in front of the hospital.

Ignoring the doctors I took Kim's hand and told him the ambulance had arrived. "We'll just get on the plane and go home. Everything is going to be all right now," I said confidently. He appeared to relax and Jill and I were both certain he understood.

The sound of the quick, efficient steps marching up the corridor and the English doctor's voice made me feel that at last someone had arrived who was capable of taking responsibility for Kim. I could now hand over and go to sleep.

There was slight consternation when the doctor realised there were two of us. He told me there would only be room for me as a passenger, I could not have a bed; Kim was the only patient he had been notified about.

He made a cursory examination of Kim and asked the Greek doctor for his diagnosis: a fractured skull with probable brain damage came the answer. At the words 'brain damage' Jill and I looked at each other questioningly, but that was something I would think about later – for the moment all that mattered was that we were going home.

The doctor dismissed the problem of getting the form signed. He said his examination had shown that Kim needed to be flown home and was in a stable enough condition to withstand the rigours of the flight; he did not need anybody to sign the forms since he was happy to accept the responsibility himself. Those words made me feel we were finally in safe hands.

Our last few minutes on Greek soil underlined my desperate wish to be off. Both of us were roughly loaded into the ambulance, with far less care than the untrained men in the pick-up truck had shown. Kim was not positioned quite correctly at first and his feet prevented the doors from being closed, so he was half dragged and half pushed further into the car. The tyres screamed as we powered out of the hospital forecourt to the airport with the siren blaring as the driver squeezed every ounce of drama from the situation. The previous thirty hours' delay made the sudden urgency appear farcical.

We screeched to a halt beside the waiting airplane on the tarmac of the tiny airport which had been specially opened for us. The official on duty decided we had to go through the proper emigration procedures and demanded our passports. I rifled through our bags searching for them while the doctor tried to convince the man that more important issues were at stake than officially stamping us out of the country; to underline his plea of urgency the airplane's engines were turning over ready to take off. But this official was not going to be diverted from his task. Finally I found the passports, he stamped them, and we could board the airplane.

When we were inside I could understand why there had been no question of taking me except as a passenger – there was no room for two horizontal patients. Squeezed into a tiny space were single seats for the doctor and nurse, a stretcher bed for Kim and a bench seat for me. In theory I could curl up and get some sleep if I wanted to, but in practice Kim's length prevented any such arrangement because his enormous feet flopped over the edge of the stretcher onto my seat, leaving me only room to sit, slightly squashed, looking out of the window.

Now I had the opportunity to relax I just wanted to put myself out for the flight. I envisaged myself surfacing gently in some hospital bed many hours hence, being told Kim was all right, then drifting in and out of sleep for a while. My dreams were shattered on two counts. First the doctor told me I would not be admitted to hospital on arrival in England because there was not much wrong with me, I would just have to go home and recover there, which frightened me terribly because it meant I had to begin to cope with life again. Secondly the tranquilliser I had been given was not having the desired effect. I craved instant oblivion but the last thirty-six hours were too deeply embedded in my mind for me to escape that easily. Every time I closed my eyes terrifying images swamped my brain, forcing me to open them again. Even reality was preferable to those nightmares.

Once we were in the air the doctor examined Kim more thoroughly and told me he was in a light coma, and although still critical he was breathing steadily, his pulse was regular and his skin colour good. He was put on a special drip which operated in spite of the atmospheric and gravitational problems in the cabin and had an oxygen mask placed over his face to help his breathing. The doctor said it was just a matter of keeping his condition stable for the rest of the flight and stopping any further deterioration so he would be able to take advantage of the facilities awaiting him in London. The outlook appeared optimistic to me.

As the plane journey progressed I began to feel everything was not under the degree of control I would have wished. The doctor seemed more concerned with impressing me with tales of his exploits than in favouring Kim with his full attention, and the nurse, who was also the doctor's wife, chatted away to the pilot oblivious of Kim's oxygen mask having fallen off his face. This was her first trip as an air ambulance nurse and I felt that recognising Kim's name had influenced her decision to respond generously to her husband's plea for help in the emergency. She seemed rather excited at dealing with someone famous, although she told me in a disappointed voice that he did not look the same as on television. She obviously felt let down by the lack of glamour on the trip – Kim was just an unconscious body, like any other.

Day was almost breaking by the time we taxied into Heathrow to be transferred into the waiting ambulance for the final leg of our journey.

The pilot told the doctor he would have to take off for Manchester, where they had all come from, within an hour or he would have exceeded his flying time and would have to take a regulation break at Heathrow. The nurse pressed the importance of getting back to Manchester and their three children, but the doctor decided that discharging his responsibilities properly meant he should travel with Kim to the hospital and personally hand him over to a doctor there.

We were loaded into the ambulance, a Ford transit type vehicle. Kim was on the stretcher flanked by the doctor and the nurse and had his drip changed from the special air ambulance type to a normal one. I was strapped into a rather rickety wheelchair, hunched under a blanket feeling like a little old lady. I watched the mild chaos around me, too tired, thankfully, to be a part of it, just an observer huddled in my granny seat.

The ambulance belonged to a private Sussex company and the ambulancemen were moonlighters from their National Health jobs, due at work later that day. They told us we had to go to the National Hospital for Nervous Diseases: they did not know where it was but once they found Oxford Circus they had directions for the rest of the journey. The doctor, sounding impressed, told me it just showed how big London was that even the ambulance crews did not know where all the hospitals were. I muttered that any London ambulance driver would know all the major hospitals but Medex had chosen people from out of town.

As I sat in the ambulance I began to feel the whole airlift was no less toytown than the thirty-six hours spent in the Rhodes hospital. Were we ever going to come across an aura of competence?

The police had apparently arranged a sort of purple corridor for the ambulance which meant we could race through London. As we sped along with the siren wailing, the second ambulanceman directed uncertainly from an A to Z atlas of London and I just hoped we were going the same route as the police expected us to take. These men had no idea of the basic geography of the city, never mind the particular location of the hospital. Meanwhile in the back of the ambulance the nurse was obviously tired and any sense of adventure about the trip had long since palled; she just wanted to get home. As she and her husband argued about the time they would eventually get back to Manchester, with her shouting about the children and him talking about his duty to the patient, the drip came out of Kim's arm and blood started spurting everywhere. I had to suppress my giggles at the black farce being played out around the inert body of Kim, who was depending on these people for his life; if I started laughing it would turn into grief-stricken hysterics.

When we finally reached the hospital the driver could find no one to greet us; in fact the hospital had given up expecting us because nobody had kept them informed about how late we were running and all the staff specially assigned to Kim had been sent home. After shuffling up and down the road from entrance to entrance I spotted a friend of mine, Pauline, and knew somebody was expecting us. The ambulance halted and she climbed in. As she put her arms round me I dissolved into loud sobs – finally Kim would be looked after properly, his survival was no longer my responsibility.

Kim's family had been at the hospital all night waiting for him: his parents, his brothers Richard and Roger, his sister Susan and her husband Paul. Kim was carried into the hospital and Susan and his mother came out to see me in the ambulance. After we had reassured each other that he was going to be all right I blurted out: "It wasn't me driving. It was him. Honest."

They both looked bemused.

"I had to tell them it was me driving because of the insurance," I explained. "But it isn't true. He was driving. I didn't do this to him."

It was ITN who had finally tracked down Kim's family, and the question of who was driving had never arisen. The family had naturally assumed Kim had been driving. I cried with relief at not having to deal with the blame and hostility of his family; it had been a nagging worry throughout the time in hospital and even during the flight. As it was I blamed myself for the accident, for not having insisted on wearing crash helmets, for even suggesting we hired bikes in the first place; that guilt was difficult enough to deal with without having other people confirm it.

I was told to go to nearby University College Hospital if I needed attention as the National had no casualty department, so Pauline climbed into the ambulance with me and we were taken there.

The doctor who examined me said there were no complications he could find and agreed it would have been better if the Greeks had not treated me at all as the Largactyl injection could have covered up any signs of concussion and the pain of the intermuscular injection was worse than the results of falling off the bike. He gave me the option of staying in overnight, but much as I longed to be looked after, I had no wish to be in a separate hospital from Kim, unable to see him, and have a rerun of the Greek situation: having to rely on other people's messages for news of his condition.

Pauline had been staying in the house while Kim and I were on holiday and she came home with me. When we finally got there the ambulance-men carried me up to my bedroom, which still had clothes strewn about it – a sign of the hurried departure for our holiday. Looking around I was vividly reminded of those hours before leaving. We had booked less than twenty-four hours beforehand, then had gone shopping for summer clothes and holiday accessories, had a friend to dinner, and at 2 a.m. had driven off to Gatwick to catch our early-morning flight. We had been so certain the holiday would put all the sadness behind us and we would return looking forward to a wonderful future. Instead Kim had survived death by sheer chance and his recovery would take months; even I would not be able to work for a few weeks.

I told myself this was not the time for thinking about how terrible things had been. The last thirty-six hours had been awful but the nightmare was over now and everything would begin getting better. I had been given Valium at the hospital and hoped that back in my own bed I could sink into a blissful sleep. Unfortunately this was impossible; every time I relaxed enough to drift into unconsciousness I was overtaken by horrendous nightmares. After a couple of hours I just gave up and went downstairs.

In the sitting-room I found a mirror and for the first time was able to see what I looked like. The sight was a shock. There was dried blood all over my forehead, including a large scab over the gash in my right temple, which looked as though it would leave a scar. Bits of encrusted blood were spattered over the rest of my face, but most surprising were the two enormous black eyes, with the bruising reaching far down to my cheeks. I resembled a wounded panda – and turned into a mournful bloodhound over the next few days as the bruising turned from blue to yellow.

The telephone rang. It was my friend Nick Davies who had heard about the accident and wanted to know if there was anything he could do. I asked him to come over and see me and drive me to the hospital to see Kim.

Nick and I had trained together in Plymouth, picked each other out on the first day, agreed to live together within a week, split up a few months later and once that side had been disposed of became very good friends. He was very fond of Kim and had been quite gooey when I gave him the news of my pregnancy. He had been our dinner guest the night before we left for Greece. He commiserated about the miscarriage and told us about his new love, Sheridan, whom he was pining for because she was on assignment for the *Guardian* in Corfu. At that time he was also on the *Guardian*, though he now works for the *Observer*.

After he had recovered from the initial shock of seeing me he was very comforting, assuring me that of course Kim would get better because life could not be so nasty for me to lose both my baby and my man in so short a time.

While we were chatting, Pauline came downstairs. When I told her of our plan to leave for the hospital immediately she cautioned me to wait a while. Her tone of voice warned me the fight for Kim was far from over. She had rung the hospital after I had been taken up to bed to check on his condition and been told he was still critical. The scan he had been given on arrival had shown his brain to be an enormous bruise. He was still in a coma but if we went along at three o'clock his consultant would meet us to give a prognosis. She had also spoken to Kim's sister, Susan, who told her that the family had stayed to hear the results of the tests and had been bleakly informed of the potential seriousness of his brain damage; his mother had said Kim would rather die than live as a vegetable and they were all naturally in a deep gloom.

As I was about to discover, off-loading responsibility for Kim had not eased my burden, only changed it. I now had to cope not just with myself but with the reactions of everybody else. While we sat and waited for the time to leave for the hospital the telephone calls began. The London media is a small incestuous world where gossip travels fast. The number of friends Kim and I had in the business, coupled with the drama of the situation, meant word had raced round and most people seemed to know about us within hours of our landing.

My friend Jilly, whom I had worked with at LBC/IRN and who had then moved on to be head of talks at Capital Radio, was the first to call. Unfortunately the news had so upset her that, far from being consoling, her shock and grief broke through the fragile reserve I had been building for myself. She asked what I had done to deserve such awful things happening to me, which was not so much a searching question as an expression of her horror at the awfulness of it all. It was more than I could deal with. I just said, "Don't say things like that," and dissolved into tears.

When I put the telephone down, Nick held me as I cried and cried. I buried my head in his chest and tears started rolling down his face as well, falling onto my hair.

He and Pauline decided that any more telephone calls could make me hysterical; I was clinging to rationality by a fraying thread which other people's clumsy sympathy could snap. My friends were wonderful people, but their common characteristic was a sense of fun, not the ability to deal with traumas well out of their experience, though they were to do their best in the coming weeks. This first day when I was still in physical shock from the accident as well as in a weak emotional state was especially bad, particularly given the problems of conveying sympathy over the telephone. Using the telephone means finding the right words, where silences are uncomfortable and have to be filled, instead of just being able to hold a hand or give a smile. I remembered some of the awkward calls of sympathy I received after my miscarriage. They had sprung from the best of intentions but once the person had said how sorry they were, I was left to try and make conversation because they were so embarrassed they did not know what else to say. I knew Pauline and Nick were right; but I felt guilty as the calls of commiseration and offers of help poured in and everybody was told I was up in bed resting.

Pauline had rung my parents, who lived in America, when we returned from the hospital a few hours earlier. I thought she had just told them what had happened and assured them I was fine, but unknown to me she had also warned them it was unlikely Kim would recover. Their return call that afternoon was one I did take.

My mother has always adopted the policy of hoping for the best but preparing for the worst and she tried to arm me for the possibility of Kim's not pulling through. I understood what she was trying to do, but for the moment I could not cope with even thinking about the possibility of his death, let alone trying to prepare myself for it. During my attempts at sleep earlier that morning I had tried to ready myself for any eventuality, but thinking of his death plunged me into such gloom that I started feeling hysterical. I decided to take a pragmatic view of the situation: as long as I was confident he would live, I felt reasonably happy and could cope, therefore there was no need to send myself over the brink by trying to prepare myself for something that might not happen. I realised that however much I tried to prepare myself for his death, if it happened it would still come as a terrible shock, and even if I was unprepared for it I would have the rest of my life to come to terms with it. Why start trying now?

I told my mother that I could not even think of Kim dying. It was obvious from my tone of voice that I was nearing the end of my personal resources for dealing with this situation. I could not bring myself to pretend any buoyancy. She offered to fly over and look after me, which I gratefully accepted, and we agreed she would arrive on Monday morning.

When we left for the hospital, I found I could not walk the short distance to the car without leaning heavily on Nick. My feet and ankles were so swollen I had to wear a pair of Pauline's shoes; luckily she had large feet. My left arm was still so painful from the injection I could not bear anyone to touch it. In the hospital, as I limped haltingly to Kim's room with my bruised and cut face, the nurses thought I looked more like a patient than a visitor.

We were asked to wait outside Kim's room because the consultant was examining him.

When Richard Hayward came out of the room he was frank but compassionate, choosing his words carefully. He stressed the gravity of the situation without causing me to become hysterical. He said Kim's condition was very serious. His brain was terribly bruised, which meant it was swollen. The skull was like a box containing it and there was enormous pressure on it, which could destroy the cells and cause brain damage. Medical technology could offer no cure for this, but the hospital had provided what he called an 'optimum environment for recovery'. Kim had been put on a ventilator which was doing his breathing for him so that the brain had as little to do as possible, thereby reducing the pressure on it. It was now up to Kim.

There was one further complication: he had developed pneumonia. He had vomited while unconscious, and in his condition one does not so much throw up as throw in and the vomit had gone into his lungs, with serious consequences. This non-smoker now had lungs like a lifelong forty a day man; I dreaded to think what the consequences would have been for a smoker.

We asked what all this meant for Kim's recovery.

Mr Hayward did not know. If things went well, Kim would start coming round in the next forty-eight hours and begin trying to pull out the ventilator tubes. If this did not happen, the consultant would have to review the situation. Further than that he was not prepared to speculate. For the moment it was a matter of waiting those forty-eight hours and seeing what transpired. Mr Hayward stressed Kim was gravely ill and still in a critical condition, but I was free to visit him whenever I wanted.

We went in to see Kim. He looked like an elephant with the ghastly contraption attached to his nose: a tube from the ventilator went down his nasal passages into his lungs. When I got over the shock of his proboscis I thought he still looked remarkably good with the deep holiday tan he had brought back with him. Lying there, his long black eyelashes resting on his cheeks, he looked peacefully asleep. Outwardly he certainly looked better than I did.

The air of competence in the room was wonderfully reassuring. He had a nurse with him all the time, who checked his temperature, pulse and reflexes every fifteen minutes. Once again he had an EEG attached to his chest, but this time it was constantly monitored.

An Australian nurse was his attendant for the day. She was happy to explain what everything was for and answer my questions about his condition. To try and convince myself that Kim was not in any real danger I said to her: "Well, he's not that bad is he? Stephen Waldorf was much more seriously injured and he's better. Stephen Waldorf was even put on a life support machine, at least Kim's not that bad."

She started laughing. "You media people. That," she said, pointing at the ventilator, "is what you call a life support machine. Stephen Waldorf was on a ventilator – most people with serious head injuries are on ventilators."

At this Nick muttered something about going for a walk. I looked up to see he had turned pale green. He hated hospitals anyway and to see a friend in this state literally turned his stomach. When he returned from his walk he looked no better, and as I was feeling dizzy and shaky myself and I knew Kim was in good hands I agreed to go home.

I felt buoyed up and optimistic from the visit until I spoke to Pauline and realised she had interpreted Mr Hayward's words as a preparation for the worst. I had realised Mr Hayward was worried, but I had seen what nobody else had – Kim's incredible strength and stamina during those critical hours in Greece when he was fighting alone with no medical assistance and still staying alive. Originally he had not even been expected to survive that first night.

But Pauline was right. The medical staff at the hospital believed Kim had deteriorated too much before he received treatment to live. If by some miracle he did survive, he would suffer from serious brain damage. They could see little hope.

Chapter 3

FIGHTING FOR LIFE

I returned from the hospital feeling physically sick and giddy and in a complete mental spin. I knew I had to sort out a plan of action for myself to survive the next few days. It was now forty-eight hours since the accident and I had not managed to have more than a few snatches of sleep lasting only minutes. I was aching all over and suffering from a booming headache. More serious was my mental condition: I was on a precipice staring into a large black hole. Every time I started to consider the possibility of Kim not making it I could feel depression immersing me; until I got some sleep and began to recover from the shock of the accident I could not trust myself to think, which meant I did not want to be left alone.

Everybody has different means of coping with crises, and I had to assess my own needs in order to keep my ability to cope. Nothing would be gained by thinking about the possibility of Kim's dying; that way lay black depression and I would be in trouble. The key to my sanity lay in believing that Kim was going to live, quite apart from the fact that if he pulled through he was going to need a lot of help from me; I had to keep myself afloat for both our sakes. The knowledge that Kim might die was of course there, but I pushed it away where it could do no harm.

Over the next few days I knew I would have to be quite ruthless in doing what was necessary to keep me relatively stable, even slightly buoyant if possible. The key to this was visitors: to have a lot of my friends coming round to cheer me up. My ploy was the right one. Entertaining gave me something to do, not physically for I could barely move out of bed, but mentally – I had to deal with people and, more importantly, their reactions to me, for they were all slightly uncomfortable.

First, everybody wanted to know what had happened and I found telling the story helped me immensely. The more I recounted it the more it became just another story rather than an awful thing that had happened to me. Some parts even made people laugh – the horrors of the Greek hospital and the scene in the ambulance were sheer black comedy. With each telling it all became less real, less upsetting. Talking about the horror became a way of not thinking about it. Ten months later a woman friend whom I had not seen since the accident asked me about it all. As I replied to her questions I became terribly upset. For the first time I could see Kim lying in the road moaning. It had been so long since I had talked about it I no longer had the story off pat and suddenly I had to think about what had happened. It was only then that I began really to come to terms with what had happened and how I had felt.

Dealing with people's shock at seeing me was easy to cope with and expected: I knew I looked appalling. My friend Jill, who had reduced me to tears on the telephone, is still mortified at the memory of her visit. She was on her way to a dinner party and called in leaving her husband in the car. She whisked into the room carrying an enormous bunch of flowers, stopped dead at the sight of me and burst into tears. She was so upset she could not stay more than a few minutes. I still have a picture of her with mascara running down her face, having to be comforted by me, telling her I was really not as bad as I looked. Other people disguised their horror rather more successfully, not that I was in the least upset by Jill's reaction; I knew her well enough to expect it.

Much more upsetting was dealing with the people who had decided Kim was not going to live. Few of them actually said anything, but my raw nerves were finely tuned and the signs were obvious. They appeared embarrassed and were slightly patronising, treating me as if I was a child, or slightly stupid, because I did not realise the truth and must be protected from the real world. I broached the subject of Kim's possible death with one of those and she told me that if Kim died it would be all right because I had a lot of good friends. I just stared at her; she did not seem to understand the difference between Kim and a friend. I knew if he died people would be sympathetic, helpful and possibly even willing to talk constantly about him for a few weeks but, as every bereaved person knows, ultimately I would be alone because only I could come to terms with it and learn to cope.

For the most part my visitors were great. I wanted to be cheered up and much of that first weekend at home I spent laughing in their company. I was grateful to everyone for trying so desperately hard to keep me going.

The person who got me through the first night after I was back was Duncan Campbell, the News Editor of *City Limits*. He has spent our friendship helping me to cope with one disaster after another. We met at my first union conference and remained friends. When we started getting to know each other he had made me feel strong enough to throw out some good-for-nothing shit whom I was allowing to walk all over me. When Kim had been sent to cover the Falklands war, Duncan considered it his duty to take me out regularly and keep me amused instead of treating me like some war widow who should sit at home and grieve, as others appeared to think. When I had my miscarriage and Kim was once again in the Falklands, Duncan came to see me in hospital and told me of three people whom he knew who had had miscarriages and now had children. He always looked on the bright side without underestimating the situation and managed to pull me round to it too.

He arrived as bright as ever, appearing to be more worried about me than disconcerted at the news. It was months later before I discovered, by chance, how he had almost broken down when he had first heard about the accident. Now, instead of talking about how devastating he had found the news he buoyed me up so I was strong enough to pull through. Like me he had great faith in Kim's ability to survive.

There were two reasons for this. The first was that his father had suffered a severe head injury when he had taken a 200 foot fall down a mountain in Glencoe, Scotland. He had been given up for dead, and was left lying overnight in a crofter's cottage. Not only did Campbell Senior survive but he managed to learn to read and write again and had recovered fully enough to take his place as a partner in an Edinburgh firm of solicitors. Now he just had a memory gap spanning a few months around the time of the accident. Secondly Duncan is an old romantic; believing that love conquers all, he had decided Kim would pull through to come back to me. There was not just me to return to: Kim did appear to be on the brink of a wonderful life with a good job, friends and everything he wanted when the accident happened.

His belief in Kim's survival made it easy for us to talk about his possible death. This made it seem less likely and the black hole receded slightly. I knew it would return when Duncan went away, but with Kim's death no longer taboo it was not quite as terrifying. Duncan's means of adding a slightly positive note to the awful prospect was to try and make me feel I was privileged even to have achieved my relationship with Kim, for however short a time; many people never found it in a lifetime. He himself had that special relationship with his girlfriend, the actress Julie Christie, so he understood that just having experienced it was a bonus. At the time I was not too sure of the logic: it was fine for him because Julie was alive and well, but I wondered what the point of having this wonderful relationship was if it was about to end – there was just that much more to miss. However, when things did appear to get too difficult and I became depressed, I did think how lucky I was to have had someone who was so special and a relationship of complete love and trust, even if it had been brief.

Duncan also told me how he admired Kim. They had first met after Kim had returned from the Falklands, when Duncan came round to do an article about Kim's experiences. Duncan had envied Kim for being sent on such a good story, but although he had admired his uncompromisingly truthful coverage he had expected to meet a conquering hero type, full of stories about his glorious exploits. Kim was certainly full of stories, but never about himself, only what he had seen and heard, the less glamorous side of army life and hilarious gossipy tales about the other journalists. There had been an immediate rapport between them.

Duncan stayed by my bed for hours that night and even tried not to leave until I had fallen asleep, understanding how terrified I was of being left alone, but I knew I would never go to sleep with him in the room, and he had made me feel good enough to fall asleep peacefully, so I made him leave.

It was a night punctuated by nightmares, but at least I got some rest. In the morning Pauline obtained an interim prescription for some tranquillisers and the promise of a doctor's visit on Monday.

In the morning Kim's brother Roger and his wife Susan came with their baby William to take me to the hospital, where I sat by Kim's bedside for a while, holding his hand and crying. Little had changed since the day before – he just lay there unconscious, breathing with the aid of a ventilator. I was there only two or three hours because I felt so wobbly I had to be taken home. His family stayed most of the day, but there was nothing any of us could do; in his coma Kim appeared oblivious of us all.

Back at home there were more visitors and the tranquillisers began to have a rather alarming effect: my tongue switched to automatic. Poor Aidan White received the full brunt of it. Aidan and his girlfriend Kate Holman had been friends of mine for years. I had met Kate when we were both doing work for the National Abortion Campaign and Aidan through the union. They were both journalists, she a freelance, he a sub-editor on the *Guardian*. I often saw Kate alone, but Aidan and I had always seen each other in company. We would go out for jokey evenings with the talk being political rather than personal; he was a friend I could count on if I was in trouble but there had never been any particularly intimate conversations between us. When I started telling him that my sex life was jinxed I could feel his embarrassment but the words kept on pouring out of my mouth. I told him that when I was first pregnant I had had terrible morning sickness, so sex was the last thing on my mind, then just as I was getting over that and beginning to feel human again, Kim was sent off to the Falklands; he came back for my miscarriage and sex was banned for ten days, then just when it was allowed again, bang, he goes and falls off a bloody motorbike. When I told him my suitcase was awash with Durex because I had bought so many for what I thought was going to be a honeymoon of a holiday he almost blushed. He managed to switch the subject, and kept the conversation firmly under control until other people arrived. I apologised when I next saw him, but he politely pretended no recollection of any embarrassment.

The next morning when I got out of bed I felt as if I was drunk on champagne. I could hardly control the use of my legs. I staggered to the loo, lurching from one wall to another and grabbing hold of the banisters as I eased my way down the stairs. I decided then that however much fun the tranquillisers might be as a temporary measure, that was all they could be: I would have to be in control if I was going to cope.

When I got to the hospital that day Kim was still unconscious, but was now breathing unaided with an oxygen mask over his nose and mouth. He had done exactly what he was supposed to do: within the allotted forty-eight hours he had started pulling at his tubes, forcing the doctors to remove them and unhook him from the machine. He had proved to everybody that against all the odds he was going to live. Days later both Mr Hayward, his consultant, and Sister Thorman, one of the ward sisters, told me they had not believed he would be able to do it. Not only were they quite frank about their prognosis being wrong, but more importantly they had ensured the care he was given was the same as if he had been expected to live. They had not allowed their opinion to dictate the standard of care and thus ensure it became self-fulfilling.

All the time Kim was unconscious I always behaved with him as if he could understand me, chattering away in my normal fashion. So when I decided to go I said goodbye to him. As I did so his eyes opened slightly and he said hoarsely: "Are you all right? Have you been terribly worried about me?"

I was so surprised I just stuttered out something trite about not worrying about me but looking after himself. He then told me he was very embarrassed about all the fuss he was causing.

By this time his family, realising he was conscious, had filed in from the corridor where they had been waiting. From behind me his mother said something, but Kim's eyes closed and his brain appeared to shut down too.

He did not say another word for two weeks, and it took months for him to regain that level of awareness and articulation. Sister Thorman told me later that she thought it had been a freak brain pattern which had surfaced, making him appear lucid when the rest of his brain was still badly damaged.

To me, standing by his bed, it was a sure sign he was going to recover fully. I thought the waiting was over. It was now just a matter of rest.

I reached home overjoyed and when I told Duncan about it he said it was typical of Kim that his first words should be concern about another person.

I must have been aware there were still a few problems in store for me, because when the doctor came round the next morning I told him I would have to have something to make me sleep, the nightmares were still dreadful, but it must leave me lucid during the day. I felt I would have a lot to cope with in the coming weeks and I knew I would have to be strong enough to keep up both my spirits and Kim's.

My mother also arrived that morning, which was wonderful because finally I had someone to take care of me, as I was able to do little for myself. She had expected to find me grieving over Kim's death, or at best to find him still in a coma, and so was very pleased to find he was going to be all right. It meant that I was in a slightly less damaged emotional condition than she had envisaged, though she still had a lot to cope with.

I am not sure that I could have managed without her. I had eaten very little in the five days since the accident, and it takes physical sustenance as well as emotional comfort to keep the spirits up. From that morning until she left it was three meals a day, cooked and brought up to me. The other major thing she achieved was to get me driving again. She drove me to the hospital once, but I was so frightened by the fact that she was obviously not quite in control that I decided even with my gammy ankle it was safer if I drove myself. To be fair, I was probably over-sensitive because of the accident, and my car's very sharp clutch combined with her being used to driving on the other side of the road and not knowing London would be enough to make anyone unsure.

When we reached the hospital on Monday the news was not good. Kim had had a relapse during the night and was back on the ventilator. I was so disappointed; I had steeled myself for slow progress, but to take a step backwards was too appalling. Over the next year I was forced to learn patience and stoicism.

When I was well enough I spent all day at the hospital beside Kim's bed. I had decided that our relationship meant I was the key person in his life – if possible he would want me there when he woke up, to tell him all that had happened, and he would want to recuperate with me. As his recovery became more prolonged I knew I was the only person who could make him pull himself through it, partly because we were so close and partly because I believed in his recovery so totally.

Understandably, his parents did not see it that way at all and my blinkered perspective was to divide us for the next year. If Kim and I had been married it would have been simpler, I would have been accepted as his primary carer, but I had chosen not to marry him. My decision had deepened Kim's mother's quite justifiable suspicion that I would leave him – in her eyes I was a temporary girlfriend.

Kim was the baby of the family and his parents felt he belonged with them. Our house was only twenty miles away from the hospital so I visited him constantly, while they lived in Bristol and had to make special journeys. Because I lived in London Kim was not going to be transferred to a local hospital in Bristol, and his parents knew that but for me they would have had him on their doorstep. The hospital accepted my slightly irregular position, partly and unfairly because of the age of Kim's parents and his father being in a wheelchair – his mother was thought to have enough on her hands.

With hindsight I should have handled the situation far more delicately and diplomatically. But all of us involved were at breaking point: the person we loved was fighting for his life. It was a time of raw emotion, not rational thinking.

I treated my visits as a working day, trying to ensure I had a friend to see at lunchtime to give me a break. For the first week Kim's sister Susan was also there, and we would spend the days sitting on either side of his bed, reading books, talking to each other and occasionally talking to him, whenever he seemed near the surface.

Every morning when I arrived I would tell him whom I had seen the night before and give him the messages of sympathy from people who had phoned or had sent either of us cards, always behaving as if he could understand because I knew hearing was the last sense to go and the first to come back. I found the number of people who cared about us quite wonderfully overwhelming. There were masses of cards and flowers sent to him at the hospital and even more arrived at home. The letters offered sympathy and occasionally practical help. I was sent bath oil to help me ease my aches and pains and offered freelance work back at IRN if I needed the money.

Every night people telephoned to find out how Kim was, all of them wishing us well. One of the most cheerful calls was from Barbara Millichip the day we arrived back from Greece. She was married to one of Kim's great friends from Birmingham, Pete. She rang to tell me that Kim was the stubbornest person she had ever met and she was certain his pig-headedness would pull him through just to prove everybody wrong.

Most evenings people came round and once I had given the daily condition report we had quite a good time. I had decided the only way to keep people coming to see me was to make their visits as pleasant as possible. I might only have been able to achieve a rather hysterical sort of happiness, obviously unreal to anyone with perception, but there was no point in an evening of misery, and general bonhomie and company did succeed in genuinely cheering me up.

One evening I came home from the hospital feeling terribly depressed.

That afternoon Sister Thorman had told me just how close Kim had come to dying. Rather than making me feel happy that he had beaten the odds and come through, it had finally brought home the horror of the first few days.

A dippy friend, Amanda Walker, came round for what was supposed to be just a few minutes because she had to get home to feed her cat Ken (named after Ken Livingstone). This was terribly important, not because poor Ken might be a bit peckish, but to give weight to Amanda's fight with boyfriend Matthew to have a baby. Matthew was rather wary about the mix of motherhood and Amanda. When Ken had been given to her he said that if she proved she could look after the kitten they would discuss having a child. (She won and they now have a daugher, Jessica.)

Poor Ken went rather hungry that night because Amanda, realising mine was the greater need, had me in tears of laughter recounting the dramatics of her discovery of what had happened to Kim and me. She did the news for the breakfast show at Capitol Radio and worked with Jill who was at home sick that day. Amanda was also feeling rather fragile because for some reason I forget she had already, in her terminology, "had a turn" about something before she reached work that morning. When she got a call from Jill dramatically ordering her not to say a word to anyone but to go into her office, close the door and take the call in there, Amanda was agog. She picked up the phone in the office to be asked by Jill if she was alone.

"Yes."

"Now sit down, Amanda, I've got some shocking news for you."

"What is it? What is it?" she cried, already near to tears.

"Calm down, Amanda. Are you sitting down?"

"Yes. Yes. What is it?"

When Jill finally told her, she had such a turn she had to be sent home for the rest of the day. She drove straight round to my house to see me, but had just sat in her car outside my house, weeping. So she scribbled a note of sympathy, pushed it through the door and went home.

The thought of her and Jill ensuring that every possible ounce of drama was squeezed from the situation just had me giggling – and I had even got Amanda a day off work. When she left I was thoroughly cheered up.

One evening Jill came round and cooked a wonderful meal, to take the burden off my mother. Amanda, not to be outdone, attempted the same a few days later. When my mother opened the door to her, she was greeted by a wail from Amanda.

"Oh, I've just had a terrible turn in the supermarket, I remembered I hate cooking. I just don't know what to do. I can't bear it."

(For my mother this was a slight improvement on their first meeting when Amanda had reeled back in horror as the door opened. Amanda, being myopic as well as dizzy, had thought it was me answering the door, having gone grey with the shock of the accident.)

My mother escorted Amanda to the kitchen and with some delicate interventions and timely suggestions guided her into producing a lovely meal.

My great need was to talk to someone who had an idea of what I was going through. My friends were all quite young and though our lives were filled with crises, normally of our own making, there were few tragedies. When I received a letter from Des Fahy who at the time presented *Weekend Reports*, the LBC programme I had worked on, I knew he was the person to talk to. His first wife, Oriel, had been killed in a car crash. I did not know the details because he never spoke of it, but I thought it likely she had died from a head injury and possibly had never regained consciousness. At first I had been reticent in contacting him in case Kim's accident brought back too many painful memories, but I took his offer of help as a sign that he would not mind talking about it.

My next problem was my inability to phone anyone: I had developed a sort of phobia about it, and could not pick up the telephone to dial a number without getting into a complete panic about having to start a conversation and talk about Kim. I did not mind people ringing me at all, but taking the initiative was just too much effort. However, I finally forced myself to pick up the phone, dial Des's number and ask for help.

Des met me at the hospital and took me out to lunch. As I started telling him what had happened I knew that he could read between the lines and know the feelings behind them. He said later he realised how fragile I felt when he saw the difficulty I had in just crossing the road: the checking, double-checking and hesitation before I was able to step off the pavement.

He told me Oriel had been killed outright and it had taken him two years to come to terms with her death, and that was only with a lot of help and support from Pam, the woman who became his second wife.

From then on every Thursday he would come to the hospital, spend some time with Kim, noting his progress, then take me out to lunch. We did not talk only about Kim and how I was coping; but he also filled me in on the latest horrors at LBC and the gossip generally.

Throughout this time Duncan would either ring or come round most evenings after doing his canvassing for the Labour Party – for these were the days running up to the 1983 general election. He managed to deal with my terrible swings of mood, my depressions, my anger, and supported my continual struggle to keep superficially happy.

One day when I was bemoaning the fact that Kim was still on the ventilator and at best only semi-conscious, he gave me his theory about Kim's lack of progress. He had decided the tremendous stamina Kim had shown during the Falklands war had been achieved by going slowly, and that was what he was doing now. Duncan reckoned that after the accident Kim had used up a tremendous amount of energy in just deciding to live; now he was resting until he felt strong enough for the next stage. I had to remember to be patient. Duncan then smiled at me: "You'd never manage to stay unconscious this long, you'd get bored and have to pop up and find out what was going on."

I began to talk about Kim a lot, particularly to my mother. I would tell her all the funny little stories about him, illustrating his idiosyncracies. I suppose I was trying to keep him alive to myself, to remember the person I had known and wipe out the reality of the body on the bed. The relationship Kim and I had had was beginning to seem illusory.

His progress was slow and erratic with many steps backwards. After the first relapse the doctors decided to take it all more slowly: he would be gradually weaned off the machine rather than be left suddenly to breathe alone. No one was quite sure what had caused the relapse; possibly his lungs were in a worse condition than had been thought and he had been taken off the ventilator before he was truly strong enough to breathe alone. So for ten minutes every hour Kim would be detached from the machine to breathe alone. He was not keen on this at all: he had obviously grown to like its doing all the work and was loath to make the effort himself. He would be hauled up into a sitting position and ordered to breathe. Every thirty seconds there would be a shouted order from his duty nurse: "Breathe!" Whoever was in the room would cajole, bully and practically force him to take a breath. I had given up smoking a year earlier, much to his delight, and I threatened to take it up again if he did not take a breath – that worked a few times. The end of the ten minutes was greeted by all of us with relief, and while he gathered up his strength for the next attempt, we tried to work out new ways of getting him to establish a breathing pattern.

I still have a vivid memory of Alison, a young, pretty Scottish nurse, who was particularly endearing because of an enormous hole in her shoe. But she was too kind, begging Kim to breathe rather than ordering him, and she received little response to her entreaties. She would push this hulking great man into a sitting position with no co-operation from him, he just sagged against her, and as she pleaded with him to breathe he would take only the odd gulp of air to keep himself alive, refusing to establish a regular pattern which would have made his breathing easier and more efficient. Kim had a penchant for women with Scottish accents and I had hoped her lovely voice would penetrate through the fog, but it seemed to have no effect.

At this stage even when conscious Kim bore little resemblance to the person I had known, he was just a body. The tube from the ventilator which passed through his nostrils down his throat and into his lungs meant he was unable to speak, and his eyes could not focus on anything for long – really he just wanted to sleep all the time.

I asked Mr Hayward again about the prognosis and he said he was optimistic, although he predicted some memory problems because the brain's memory bank is behind the left temple, where Kim had taken the fall. The speech part of the brain is there too, but Mr Hayward was not worried about that because he had heard about Kim talking to me and had also seen for himself. When he had said good morning to Kim, Kim had mouthed good morning back. The nurses and I thought he was just sucking up because he certainly would not respond like that to any of us lesser mortals. Mr Hayward mentioned that Kim could have problems for a long time and gave as an example that Kim could find himself in a shop but completely forget what he had gone in there to buy. As Kim's memory was anyway fairly dreadful, particularly in circumstances like that, I could not see life changing very much. At the time I had no idea what a crippling disability a severe memory problem is.

I was managing some basic communication with Kim during this time:

he could make simple hand signals and one could tell a lot from the expression in his eyes. He would give me the thumbs up or thumbs down when I asked him a question and could slightly nod or shake his head. With hindsight I do not know how much he did understand or how often he was kidding me by nodding; he could have just been trying to respond correctly to please me, as he did quite often later on. I did not demand too many responses and mostly kept up a monologue when he was awake: the thumbs up or down were usually used to indicate whether he wanted me to go on talking or shut up, and he was quite capable of making it clear when he wanted me to stop talking.

I do not know whether he really knew or remembered all the people I would chatter about, but there were two instances which made me certain that on occasions he could understand completely.

The first time was when I was discussing with one of the nurses how much he would remember of our relationship, wondering if we would have to start all over again. To find out I asked him if he remembered I was rather bossy. He rolled his eyes so expressively I started giggling; it was the visual equivalent of, is the Pope a Catholic?

I received the same response when I was talking to him about the FA Cup Final. In my attempt to keep him up to date with the latest sporting news, which I knew was important to him, I would faithfully relate all the latest scores and happenings in subjects far from my heart like football, cricket and even rugby. The 1983 Cup Final had ended in a draw after extra time, causing a replay. I was telling him about it but he did not seem particularly interested so, wondering if he was following me at all, I asked him if he knew what the FA Cup was. I received That Look in reply, which also indicated hurt that I could even ask the question. Friends later told me his disinterest was probably because he was not keen on either of the teams, mixed with slight disbelief at any pronouncements I made about sport.

When his sister Susan returned to her family in Winchester I began to get to know his nurses. During the hours that Kim slept we would chat away about their problematic love lives and about the hospital and nursing in general. I was shocked by the hours they worked and the responsibility they had in relation to their paltry salaries. The most striking thing about the nurses was their youth: the two women in charge of the ward, Sister Kennedy and Sister Thorman, were only in their mid-twenties and were running a ward full of acutely ill people, while the staff nurses who looked after Kim were barely out of their teens. They did the dreary job of keeping him clean and washed and continually clearing the tube coming out of his nostrils up from his lungs, and throughout this tedious work they had to keep ever vigilant for signs of impending danger; something not spotted in time could have fatal consequences. On one particular bad day on the ward, when every unconscious patient seemed to have dirtied himself and the air smelt foul, one of the nurses turned to me and said: "This job is just shovelling shit."

When it looked as though Kim was finally getting his breathing sorted out he had a second relapse. Nobody could understand what the matter was or what had happened, but once again he was back on the ventilator full time, with the weaning process even more gradual.

Fifteen days after the accident it happened again. When I arrived in the morning I was asked to wait outside his room in the corridor. He had vomited earlier that morning so forcefully that it had splattered all over the wall a few feet away from the bed, and then he had collapsed; again he was relying on the ventilator literally as a life support machine. Tests were being done to try and ascertain the cause of the relapses; his blood gas levels had been checked, he was having a thorough physical examination and he was booked in for a brain scan.

Later Sister Thorman told me how serious the relapse had been. After Kim had been sick and was back on the ventilator, the nurse looking after him called her into the room because Kim was turning blue. Although he was attached to the ventilator, which should have been breathing for him, he was suffocating; she had to get a pair of bellows to force the air into his lungs and make him breathe so he would live.

Poor Sister Thorman, it was not one of her better days. Later that morning one of the patients in the big male ward started throwing trolleys around the room, narrowly missing Samer, a fellow patient who could not move, speak or seemingly understand, though his eyes showed terror as the trolley came towards him. She calmed the assailant down, chastising the huge man like a naughty child, knowing it was all bluff for she would have been as easy to pick up as the trolley. Two male porters were called to take him away to a ward where he could be restrained and not endanger other patients.

That afternoon Eamon was admitted. It was thought he had been mugged, but nobody knew how, where or why because there were no witnesses and even the person who had telephoned the ambulance had disappeared by the time it arrived. He was in a critical condition with a serious head injury and appalling internal injuries.

I was sitting in the corridor when his family arrived to ask about his condition. I could hear Sister Thorman trying to prepare them for the worst; she was giving them the facts and leaving her opinion out of it, but her voice showed she did not think he was going to make it. I realised that was how people had spoken to me, but I just had not wanted to hear it.

Eamon's arrival meant Kim had to be moved from his single room into the main ward, for there were not enough staff on duty at night for them to have a nurse each, while in the main ward they could be put in next door beds and one nurse could care for the two of them. I was witnessing the practical effects of the Health Service cuts and learning that the argument that they only affected non-urgent cases was a myth. The ward appeared to be operating on a skeleton staff throughout Kim's stay, though after he left there were yet further reductions.

When Sister Thorman went off duty that afternoon, after a few more minor crises, she came into Kim's room to say goodbye and give his condition a final check, as she did every day. She sat down on his bed, put her hands on his shoulders to force him to pay attention and said: "Kim Sabido, you have let me down today. It has been awful and so have you. I want to see you up and about and helping me very soon."

The whole time he was on the ventilator she treated him as if he could understand, bullying him, cajoling him and encouraging him to get better. He says he does not remember his stay at Queen's Square at all, but whenever he sees Sister Thorman his face always lights up, though he has no actual memories of her.

I had not seen him at all that morning when I went out to lunch with Des, feeling rather depressed at the thought of watching Kim begin all over again for the third time, and wondering just how long it was going to be before he did manage to get off the ventilator and begin the process of recovery. On my return from lunch he was still undergoing tests so Des and I went for a walk.

It was late in the afternoon before I managed to see him, by which time Louise was the nurse looking after him. She was one of the few nurses on the ward whom I had never met. Her brother had been in a submarine during the Falklands war, so she knew who Kim was and had heard some of his despatches: not that she was at all in awe of him as she demonstrated during the rest of his stay, but she did have a special interest in him.

She was very keen on upholding the dignity of patients; whether unconscious or supposedly a vegetable she thought they should be accorded the treatment a normal adult would expect. But what made me so grateful to Louise was her theory about why Kim was not getting any better.

She told me that there appeared to be nothing the matter with him apart from a high temperature, yet he could no longer survive without the ventilator, and even his temperature, which was coming down, had no apparent cause. Not one of the battery of tests had come up with the slightest clue to his malaise.

To demonstrate the problem she detached him from the ventilator; he made no attempt to take a breath, even with the two of us shouting at him. She had to reconnect the tube to get him to start breathing again.

She asked me what he was usually like when he was ill, with coughs and colds and the like. I told her he was dreadful; he made an enormous fuss, took lots of medicine and went into such a decline of misery he was quite unpleasant to be with. She suggested this was the cause here, he was indulging his illness and letting himself be overcome by it.

At first I was quite cross. This was no trivial complaint, he had nearly died; it seemed grossly unjust to accuse him of hypochondria.

Louise repeated that nothing could be found wrong with him and whereas a minor ailment will still go away if one allows oneself to succumb to it, in this case it would not. He had become addicted to the ventilator and did not want to live without it; because he had been on it so long he had to make a conscious effort to start breathing on his own again, and for the moment he was finding it easier to let the machine do the work.

Louise thought he was malingering.

I went home and thought about what she had said. I dressed it up more romantically but basically came to the same conclusion.

I was no longer sure he even wanted to live. I felt it had taken so much effort to pull through at the beginning that he had no energy left. He still appeared to be in the strange land of half-life and half-death, drifting in and out of consciousness, barely knowing what was real and what was part of his dreams and imagination.

My mother had told me that after my second major kidney operation, when I was eight, my father had visited me in hospital the next day. When he asked me how I was I turned weakly towards him and told him I felt so awful I wished he had just let me die.

I do not remember the incident and am now thankful I did have the operation and am alive, but I thought that perhaps Kim was going through the same sort of experience. Living was just too tough, dying seemed so much more pleasant, and this half-world he inhabited at the moment would do fine until he made up his mind.

Remembering how the dreams of a deep, deep sleep appear more real than anything outside, I thought he might not be aware of what his options were. Possibly he did not understand that to be with me, his family and his friends he had to come back to life; since we must have been part of his dreams maybe he thought we were living with him in his funny little world.

I decided to try and pull him out of it because I was beginning to doubt that otherwise he would survive. I had relied on both his physical and mental stamina to bring him out of the coma, but if he had given up maybe he would not live after all, or he would spend months on the machine before he got bored and made the effort to re-enter the real world. I had a partial experience of how keen he was on the unconscious world from trying to wake him up on days when he was not working; when he knew there was no need to be awake he preferred to sleep.

The next day I was going to talk to him.

When I arrived that morning Louise was once again by Kim's side. (I was learning about the terrible shifts done by nurses.) I told her of my plan and she agreed it could do no harm and might even achieve something.

I waited until Kim became aware of my presence, told him I had something important to say and asked him if he was listening, to which he gave the thumbs up.

I began by explaining my theory to him, about why I thought he might have doubts about wanting to live. Then I told him I needed him and desperately wanted him to live. I was finding it terribly lonely without him and was having awful problems sorting out all the affairs of the house and gently reminded him that he had taken on all the paperwork because I was so hopeless at that side of things and now the house seemed awash with unanswered letters and unpaid bills. I told him I was missing him terribly because visiting this mute person in hospital was no substitute for having the real thing back at home. I said that although he might believe I was in his funny little world with him, I was not, I was here in the real world, the unpleasant painful world, and if he wanted to be with me he would have to come back to it. I explained that I knew it would be an enormous effort, very painful and hard work, but that was what it was going to take to live again. He had to be independent of the machine, to breathe alone, that was the first step in beginning to live; it could no longer be a gradual process, he should not allow himself to be passively weaned off it but must take charge and actively pull himself off it. He had to start fighting the machine.

I went on in this vein for some time. At the end I asked him if he had understood. He nodded and then appeared to sink back into his normal stupor.

My lecture seemed to have had no effect; hardly surprising, I suppose, but I was disappointed nevertheless.

Three hours later he started fighting the machine. The dials showed he was no longer allowing the ventilator to breathe for him, but trying to do it alone. When he was unhooked for a few minutes he needed no encouragement to breathe. He was taking short sharp gasps rather than slow, deep breaths, so he could not keep it up for long alone, but at least he appeared to have taken control.

Louise and I felt quite pleased with ourselves.

As Kim grew alert he started trying to communicate with us, but because he could not talk we had no idea what he was trying to say. That Friday afternoon Susan came to visit and both of us desperately tried to understand Kim's mouthings – as the tube down his nose into his lungs prevented any sound from coming out. We gave him a piece of paper and a pencil but he could not write anything that made sense. Remembering that Duncan's father had had to relearn how to read and write, I wondered if it would be the same for Kim. In his big letters, on a piece of card, I wrote KIM and asked him what it said. He immediately mouthed his name and then, in case we had not understood, pointed to himself. Susan and I printed our own names on the paper, but that was not so successful; however, at least I knew that Kim could not only understand what was being said to him but could also read. I thought he balked at our names because he was bored of the game. Later I found out he had no idea what our names were.

The nurses and physiotherapist had some doubts about how much he could really understand and how much he was pretending to, because he seemed to nod his head to most questions. In retrospect I think they were right. There were times when he would switch off and not listen, but to try and please everybody he would nod his head at what appeared to be the appropriate moments. But there were also times when he was lucid. That afternoon when the physiotherapist came in to bang his back and make him cough, as she did twice a day while he was on the ventilator as his lungs became congested, for the first time he started being unco-operative and not doing as he was told. She told him, laughing, that he was just a troublemaker, so he turned to her and smiled, then gave an eerie cackle. She came over to me and told me he was going to be trouble when he was able to move and talk.

It was another sixty hours before he had the tubes pulled out of his lungs and was finally free of the machine. During that time he fought it steadily. As he became increasingly alert and aware of his environment he began trying to pull the tubes out himself. We discovered just how strong his hand grip and arms were as his sister Susan, the nurses and I all tried to keep him from pulling out his tubes.

The others also kept telling him to relax when the machine was switched on, to stop fighting it and let it breathe for him; of course I could not because I had told him to start fighting it in the first place.

I do not know whether my pep talk did any good at all, whether Kim understood it or was even listening. It could have been sheer coincidence that he picked up after it, but Louise and I are convinced it did the trick. I was probably being melodramatic worrying about him not living, and he would have pulled through anyway, but it could have taken a lot longer.

The next day Joan Thirkettle, a reporter with Kim at ITN, came in with a tape she had made up for him. She had spent the week going around ITN getting everybody who knew him to record a message encouraging him to get better. The tape was wonderful and although that day Kim did not have the concentration to take it in and really understand what he was listening to, he played it to himself many times in the ensuing months, each time amazed at how many people cared. Many of the messages were private jokes, with the people on the Foreign Desk promising him wonderful trips or threatening a return to the Falklands, and one of the news editors threatening to put him back on a story which had been the bane of his life for the weeks before he was sent to the Falklands. Jon Snow begged him to come back because he could not keep the revolution going without him, and there were an awful lot of women, whose names and voices I did not recognise, telling him that lunches were not the same without him.

The tape had reached the ears of the *Sunday Mirror* and they ran a story on him, so on the Sunday I took in a copy of the paper to show Kim. Disappointingly he did not appear to understand that this was a story about him with his picture in it. He would not even try to read it.

That weekend was terribly frustrating because there was so much to say to him, but I was never quite sure how much he was understanding. For the first time he appeared to be Kim again, which made the lack of communication even more difficult. When his niece Claire came to visit him I hoped she might be able to interpret his mouthings, as she is deaf and can lip read. But she just shrugged her shoulders, perplexed. She was only eleven and very fond of her youngest uncle; seeing this strange thing in bed with tubes coming out of his nose may have been too much for her. Or was Kim just talking nonsense?

There were so many questions which could only be answered when he was off the ventilator and communicating properly again.

Chapter 4
AMNESIA

On Spring Bank Holiday Monday, nineteen days after the accident, I arrived at the hospital bubbling with excitement and expectation.

Kim had been taken off the ventilator during the night, so finally the waiting was over. After three and a half weeks I could have my boyfriend back. Now he no longer had the tube down his throat stopping him from speaking, everything would be all right again.

I could spend the morning filling in the gaps in his memory for him. He was probably even rather confused about why he was in hospital as it was unlikely he remembered the accident, but it was just a matter of clearing that up, explaining what had happened and then he would soon be home for a long, slow convalescence.

It would be so good just to talk to him again. The past few weeks had not only been a strain because of the constant worry, I had also missed him as confidante and adviser. I had been used to talking to him every day, having him constantly there to turn to, to discuss everything with from political scandal to domestic trivia. Three weeks with only the odd hand signal or facial expression had been hell. I needed him back, accepting that he would be physically weak and tire easily, just to have him to talk with.

I rushed into the ward and waved to Kim in bed, but was immediately shooed out because the doctors were doing their rounds.

Ten minutes later when I was allowed back in, Kim was no longer in his bed. Hunched in the armchair beside it was a bent, gaunt figure, an old man with blank dark eyes, one of which could not focus, staring out of an emaciated face. Kim looked like the pictures of people released from Belsen and Auschwitz, a skeleton barely covered by skin and those dead eyes indicating no working thought processes behind them.

I do not know whether the rose-tinted spectacles had been pulled from my eyes and I was finally seeing Kim as everybody else had been seeing him, or whether because I had been with him every day I just had not noticed him physically wasting away and it was only now he was out of bed that the dramatic weight loss was so apparent.

When I bent to kiss him I realised it was not just physical deterioration. He was blank. I said his name and asked how he was, and he smiled back, but only just, and whispered something unintelligible. Even raising his head to look at me was obviously a strain.

I felt as if I had been kicked in the stomach. It was the death of my expectations. This was no companion sitting in front of me, more a zombie. As long as the tube had prevented him speaking I had been able to fool myself that everything was fine and our communication difficulty was due to that. I now saw for myself that the problems went far deeper.

I was to learn that every significant advance, and coming off the ventilator was certainly that, carried with it a kick in the teeth; every bit of progress brought with it new evidence of the injury for me to come to terms with.

Later that morning I learned that Kim had tried to follow me when I had first been hustled out of the ward; he had got out of bed but had collapsed at the first step because his legs were not strong enough to carry his weight – so somewhere in there he did know I meant something to him.

The thought that he had recognised me kept me going, as I was finally forced to accept the reality staring me in the face. He could hear what was said to him, see what was going on around him and apparently understand, but the responses were on the level of an automaton. He would raise his right hand if requested, nod if I asked him whether he was tired when his eyelids began to droop or if he wanted me to plump up his pillows or wind up the bed so he could sit up easily as he restlessly fidgeted. He was now physically able to speak, but could manage no more than a word or two at a time, and always in a whisper because of the terrible sore throat the tubes had given him. As I sat there with him it was difficult to see the Kim I had known and loved.

I asked myself if this was what a cabbage was. I wondered if my idea of an inert form only technically alive was a misconception. Perhaps Kim's brain would never properly come back into use again; it was possible that while the motor functions were largely unimpaired, the intellectual part was irreversibly damaged. Had we all been through the last few weeks to be left with someone who was alive enough to make demands, but was not a whole person? Was this the price that I had to pay for my determination that Kim would live? It seemed rather like the wishes that are made in fairy-tales, which are granted in such a way one regrets ever having made them.

As I sat with Kim I was not prepared to accept that the battle to save his life had been merely a Pyrrhic victory. But was there a person inside the befuddled brain trying to get out? Did the real Kim exist or had he died in the crash, leaving just this body?

For me there was only one answer possible: I had to believe there was hope. This was not my boyfriend but he was in there somewhere and I was going to get him back. The nurses had tried to warn me this would happen when he came round, but not only had I not wanted to hear, I had genuinely been unable to understand what they were trying to tell me. Like most people, I had no idea of the shades of grey in the problem: to me, people were either all right or they were inert cabbages. I was to learn that between these two extremes is a whole spectrum of disabilities of varying degrees.

The nurses reassured me that most people were confused when they came off the ventilator, because of the drugs they had been given, and one of the reasons for his unresponsiveness was exhaustion. He had hardly had any sleep the night before as he fought against the ventilator and there had been the constant struggle with the nurses as he tried to pull out his tubes. Finally they had conceded to the inevitable, and at four in the morning had hauled both an anaesthetist and physiotherapist out of bed to remove the tubes and bang his chest so he would be able to breathe alone. A night like that would have exhausted most people, let alone someone in his physical condition. It was another display of his stubborn, unrelenting willpower.

It was the memory of those words he had spoken when he first regained consciousness that gave me confidence he would recover. He had known what was going on, been perfectly lucid and sure who he was talking to. I decided it was impossible for him to have mentally deteriorated since he came into hospital, so he might be in a relapse but he would definitely return to that level, and that was the Kim I knew. That memory was to keep me going for months, because in spite of constant improvement, progress was painfully slow. It was often difficult to imagine he would ever be just an ordinary person with whom I could have normal conversations, instead of someone who constantly needed special care and attention and for whom allowances always had to be made.

Nobody else took my theory seriously and the optimism was quite possibly built on an entirely false premise, but that unflagging certainty of a complete recovery stopped me sinking into despair as I faced the frustrations of the ensuing months and, more important, it meant I never allowed Kim to doubt he would get better.

In spite of the cheerful front I kept up with Kim that day and my determination that there would a happy ending, I sank into depression when I returned home. Could someone in his state really ever get back to 'normal'? I promised myself that if he did recover I would write a book, so that anybody else going through what I had been through that day would know there could be light at the end of the tunnel.

The next day my mother came in with me. She was leaving for America the following morning and wanted to say goodbye to Kim. He did not appear to recognise her – hardly surprising as they had seldom met – but he was extremely polite. Sitting delicately in his armchair, still with the movements of an old man, he offered her a hand in greeting, said hello and gave her a little smile. He nodded as she reminisced about the last time they had met but nothing sparked, so it appeared more a matter of good manners than reviving memories. As she left he whispered goodbye.

The visit left her optimistic. She had been an occupational therapist and for some time had worked with people who had had strokes, teaching them how to communicate. She felt that even Kim's muted conventional responses showed an awareness of how one was supposed to behave in that social situation and therefore a functioning brain.

After the ventilator tubes were removed Kim still had three tubes attached to him: a drip into his arm, a feeding tube into his nose and a catheter for his urine. His victory over the ventilator left him with no patience for these. By the second day he had forced a nurse to remove the food tube, otherwise he would have pulled it out himself, having done just that to his drip. This left only the catheter which he also hated but posed rather a dilemma, for the more pulled at it the more he hurt himself as it was fixed inside his penis. Now that he was fully conscious there was no medical reason for having it there but it saved the mess and bother if he was incontinent. As he continued to fiddle with it, refusing to be distracted from his task of pulling it out even though it was beginning to cause some bleeding, the nurses decided to let him have his way and removed it for him.

I explained to him that when he wanted to go to the loo now he must ask me or a nurse for a bottle, but he never did. It meant taking the initiative instead of just responding to questions or commands and this was too much to ask of Kim. It also offended his natural modesty; his bodily functions were private and not something he wished to talk about. Not once, to my knowledge, did he ever ask for a bottle, it was always a matter of second-guessing him; and if the nurses and I failed there were the consequent wet pyjamas. Within two days he could walk, with help, to the loo, and do his doings in private, but even then he would just say he wanted to go for a walk, and I would have to ask whether he wanted to go to the loo, to which he would either respond with a nod or say no, he just wanted to go for a walk.

The most significant event of that second day off the ventilator was the visit of Kim's friend Andrew Burn from Birmingham. I had asked him to come down because I felt that just having me and his family as companions could be getting rather claustrophobic for Kim, and perhaps by now he was needing a bit of 'boys' talk'. My attempts to keep him up to date with all the latest sporting gossip were a bit phoney; he knew how little I cared about the latest triumphs and disasters in the footballing world, and attempting any kind of analysis was quite beyond me, while Andrew talked of little else. Kim and Andrew had gone to watch the Wales-England rugby match in Cardiff earlier in the year, and when they had returned I asked Kim what they had talked about all day. He told me that before the match they had talked about possible results and plays, and afterwards they had talked about what had happened compared to what should have happened.

Andrew's girlfriend Julie had travelled down from Birmingham with him, but we agreed Andrew would see Kim alone; not only was it probable that Kim would not recognise Julie, but he could not deal with more than one person at a time, and then his moments of concentration were few and far between. Being with Kim was rather like sunbathing in

England: a long wait for the sun to come out from behind the clouds, then a brief interval of basking in its rays.

Julie walked into the ward with Andrew, just to wave hello. Seeing the sudden shock on their faces brought a lump to my throat. As Andrew quickly pulled himself together, smiled, held out a hand and said, "Hello, Tonto" (Kim's Birmingham nickname), I could feel my eyes filling up.

In the corridor Julie and I, both feeling rather embarrassed, wiped our eyes. She had known it was going to be a shock seeing Kim, as I had carefully explained his condition to Andrew, but nothing could prepare her for the shock of seeing this person who was no longer the man she knew.

Afterwards Andrew said that once he had got over the initial shock of seeing this emaciated being in the bed he found the visit quite easy. He adjusted himself to the rhythm of choosing a topic, rambling on in a monologue for a few minutes as Kim nodded, then, when Kim's attention flagged, changing the subject. When Kim switched off in a doze, Andrew just read one of the rugby magazines he had brought down as a present.

Running out of topics, Andrew started telling Kim about the plans to have professional rugby games on the same lines as the Kerry Packer cricket circus. This had been the big news on the sports pages for the last few days, and as he plunged into details of the reactions and general whys and wherefores he realised he was making it all far too complicated for Kim's limited concentration span. Even if he had begun by following the account he must have lost the thread by now, but not wanting to stop in mid-stream Andrew continued until he felt he had properly explained every aspect.

When he had finished, Kim leaned over to him and hoarsely whispered: "Well, you needn't worry about them wanting you."

Andrew looked up stunned, then realising he had heard right, replied: "You cheeky bugger."

Kim just grinned.

When Andrew told me the story I knew for certain Kim was in there and was going to come back.

My daily arrival at the hospital was always greeted by a catalogue of

Kim's antics from the nurses. The next morning Louise told me how they had been walking him to the loo when he had veered off in the direction of a newly-made bed. He pulled out his penis, and just in time she realised what he was about to do. Thinking of her clean sheets she spun him round, so instead he peed all over her shoes. Luckily she just roared with laughter. She did the same when he squirted shaving cream all over her face; she was just delighted he was showing some spirit.

The next morning Scottish Alison was helping him to the loo when he stubbed his toe. He sank dramatically to the floor and raising his eyes to Alison he whispered a word she could not quite catch. Thinking it could be something important she bent down to ask him what he had said.

"Ouch," he said, with enormous eyes giving him an air of complete melancholia.

I thought the story was very funny, it was so good to know his hypochondria had returned. The day before the accident he had tripped over and fallen on his knee. His agonised writhings were met with my normal sympathetic response: convulsions of giggles. When we had both recovered he sternly pointed out the serious complications that could arise from a knee injury, such as the cartilage falling out.

That morning in hospital I was quite sure Kim would have told Alison about the possible dire consequences of a stubbed toe if he had had more control over his vocabulary, but he had to be content with 'ouch'.

As he gradually improved over the next few days he slowly started to make sentences, and I began to get more out of him than just a 'yes' or a 'no'. The best way to get a response was to be rude to him. One evening when he considered I had gone quite far enough he told me to "go away, you beastly old pig". I felt this was great progress.

Physically he was becoming much stronger and it was obvious he was concentrating all his energy into getting himself independently mobile again, while his intellectual capabilities were just being allowed to develop slowly.

His attempts at walking were a tragi-comic spectacle: this enormous gangling man, like a daddy long-legs, desperately trying to put one foot in front of the other without buckling under his own weight, being propped up by a tiny nurse on either side. Within two days he was unstoppable. He would do circuits round the men's ward unaided, saying hello to everyone, then when he found this boring he would go across to the women's ward where he was a great hit. When I was there I would try and go with him, to make sure he did not get into trouble, bother people or get lost, but I found the constant exertions exhausting. He was for ever being brought back by some poor nurse as I sat worn out in the chair beside his bed. The problem was that Kim still needed constant attention, but very little of it medical. The nurses on the understaffed ward just did not have the time for him, as they had other patients with far more pressing needs. Allowing me to disregard visiting hours and see Kim all day was not just a kindness to me but a virtual necessity just to keep him out of trouble.

His determination to get himself back into shape physically led to our first row. In the first few days of being able to walk he had lots of drive and energy but little direction or balance. He kept on wanting to walk up and down the ward to get it right, and he was probably bored just lying in bed with me for company. By early evening I was becoming exhausted from supporting his weight during his constant totterings and wanted to call a halt. Without supervision the ward was not a safe place for him to walk because there were many seriously ill people with the attendant drips and machines beside their beds to be bumped into or knocked over. Kim's constant perambulations were beginning to get on the nurses' nerves as they continually had to remove obstacles from his random paths, and it was an evening when a lot of medical problems cropped up.

When I suggested stopping for the night Kim shook his head and just got up to indicate that alone or accompanied he was going to walk. When I tried to stop him he was so angry that his voice almost returned to its normal level.

He told me to "Fuck off, you old cow."

I was too tired and emotionally involved to argue with him and I was anyway not quite sure whether it would end with me in giggles or tears, so I accompanied him for another round of the ward. When we met Louise I explained the problem to her. She suggested to him that he rest for a bit because everybody was busy and he was getting in the way. He made the mistake of swearing at her.

She propelled him across the ward, giving him a lecture on manners, and pushed him down into the armchair beside his bed.

"We are all much too busy to keep an eye on you as well as people who are really ill," she told him. "Now you just sit there quietly and behave yourself. If you try getting out of your chair we will tie you into it."

With that she marched off.

Poor Kim. He was like an inflatable toy after being pricked with a pin. He was almost in tears. I had to try and cheer him up, telling him she had not meant to be nasty, but everybody was too busy for him at the moment. When Louise next passed his bed I called her over so he could apologise to her. She realised she had upset him and told him not to worry about what he had done, so he was slightly cheered up.

One characteristic of Kim's which did not seem to be returning was his appetite. Living with Kim had been a good way of making sure no food was wasted: he would eat everything on his plate and then anything I had not been able to manage. Once, when staying with my mother, as she handed him his third heaped helping of the main course she said weakly she did not think she had got enough food in for the weekend. I had to point out to her that Kim would go on accepting more as long as he was offered it, but did not notice if he was not given a chance to have a second helping. He had an almost Pavlovian response to any offer of food: instant acceptance.

His body had never reflected the amazing quantities he gobbled, though there had been some extra padding around the midriff which I was always complaining about and urging him to lose. When I saw his emaciated figure I swore I would never complain again about him being overweight, a promise I broke as soon as his figure returned to normal.

In those first two weeks I was worried because Kim seemed to be barely eating at all; he had no interest in food. Given what was produced by the hospital this was quite understandable, but he had never seemed bothered by quality before.

On his first day of being able to eat he was given a plateful of liquidised mush: a clump of green, a clump of orangey white and a clump of brown, presumably all adding up to meat and two veg. That evening he was allowed solids – fish, chips and peas. It had been cooked hours before, the batter of the fish was so tough I had difficulty cutting it up for him, the chips were congealing fast and the peas were solid. With a lot of coaxing he ate almost half.

I did not understand why someone in his condition, who had just come off what was, in effect, a three-week fast, was not given more appetising and nutritious food. I felt he should have been on a special diet to build him up. During Kim's stay he was presented with a succession of overcooked, boring, bland dishes. Hospitals are about getting well, yet healthy eating seems to be discouraged with fresh fruit and vegetables a rarity, carbohydrates served up three times a day, and whatever goodness might have been in the food originally relentlessly boiled out.

Luckily for Kim it did not take him long to regain his appetite and revert to his old habit of demolishing anything put in front of him. Long-stay patients who are more particular eaters seem to have to rely on their visitors for their nutrition.

At the end of the week Kim's parents came up to see him. Over the five days there had been the most remarkable improvement. He could now walk, though he dragged his right foot because his brain damage meant he was still not fully in command of the right side of his body. The other obvious physical problem was his wandering eye. Though he still spoke in a whisper his responses showed more awareness of what was being said to him and what was going on around him. But his parents had not watched the improvement, they had not seen him since he lay unconscious like a sleeping prince waiting for his princess, looking as though when he woke everything would be all right. They were terribly shocked at the state of him, finding it difficult to see the bits of Kim glimmering through this mockery of him, the signs which pointed to the potential of the future, and they could not share my optimism. There had been too many tragedies in that family for them to have acquired my naive belief in happy endings.

It was still extremely difficult having a conversation with Kim because he had almost no working memory. He could not remember his childhood, what had happened yesterday or even what had happened fifteen minutes ago. So he could not answer questions because he knew no answers and rarely attempted to initiate a conversation because he could not think of anything to say. The stereotype of an amnesia victim wandering around perfectly normally, understanding daily life but just not knowing his identity, bears little relation to memory problems due to brain damage. Kim's memory was so bad he would forget what he was trying to say before he had finished saying it. His lack of memory made it impossible to gauge his intellectual ability. His father particularly found it terrible to see Kim in such a state.

The two days of his parents' visit left everybody physically and emotionally exhausted, but for the first time Kim had to deal with people's demands and it brought him one step nearer real life. With anybody else he switched off as soon as he began to get tired, but he knew how much his parents cared and needed reassurance that something was working in his brain, and he did his best to respond. It was wonderful seeing how much effort he made and seeing that the potential for that effort was there. In many ways his parents' visit woke him up from the little world he retreated to.

He told his brother Roger, who had driven his parents up from Bristol, that he felt he was in prison. And it was true, a mental prison with his own brain providing the bars and an indefinite sentence. His consultant Mr Hayward gave the analogy of a heavy door having been slammed shut on his mind. Now it was a matter of prising it open bit by bit; but it was up to Kim to open that door, and to do it he had to use the very part that the door was closed upon, his mind.

An hour or so after Kim's parents had left, one of the nurses did his regular four-hourly check. As well as taking his temperature and pulse, the procedure was to ask him the date and where he was, to gauge his orientation. Often the nurse would stay and ask a few more questions or attempt to have a chat with him, which was always more constructive because he never had a clue about the data or where he was: it was to be weeks before there was a chance of an intelligent answer to either question. This time she asked him a few questions about himself. He knew his name but little else.

When she had left he turned and asked me why people always asked him questions. I told him they were trying to get him to remember his life before the accident. He said he did not want to remember it. I was surprised and asked why.

"Because it was horrible."

I was shocked. "No it wasn't, Kim, you had a wonderful life before the accident. You had lots of friends, you were terribly happy, you had a good job – you were a reporter at ITN. Most people would envy that life."

"Will you tell the nurses that please?"

"They all know that, some of them have even seen you on television."

"They act like I'm nothing."

I tried to reassure him and took him to Sister Thorman so that he could tell her the problem and she could try to deal with it. But there was no easy solution because having no idea of who he was or what he had done he had nothing on which to base any self-respect or confidence.

When Kim was off the critical list he was allowed as many visitors as he liked, and now he was able to speak people wanted to come and see him, which I thought was a good idea, particularly after his reaction to the nurse's question. His family did not share this view wholeheartedly. They felt he would not want people to see him in his rather moronic state and would be embarrassed about it when he got better; they also felt he could become the object of ridicule and he might be humiliated by visitors. I knew Kim would be just as embarrassed at his parents having seen him in this state, if not more so, and there were more important points at issue.

A relatively easy way to get Kim to recall his past was for it to be literally paraded in front of him: a protracted *This Is Your Life*. For this he needed his friends to jog his memories, because the part of the past he would have difficulty with was not his childhood spent at home – early life is so firmly imprinted on the brain it is almost impossible totally to eradicate – but the ten years since he had left the family fold.

Kim also needed stimulation which the medical staff could not provide: people to talk to, to force him to push himself mentally as far as he could go. I could not do this alone because I had neither the energy nor the ability to be constantly fascinating. His friends could supply different sorts of stimulation, with their own personality dictating individual approaches filling in various parts of his past, fuelling his interests.

In fact there was never a choice. I could not have kept people away even if I had wanted to. There were so many who wanted to see him.

At first they did tire him out and he would shut his eyes after a few minutes to indicate he had had enough, but as he grew stronger they became a vital part of his life, and he would feel quite unhappy if an hour went by without somebody coming to see him. Any fears about people coming to laugh at him or upsetting him by not being able to cope with his condition were quickly dispelled. Although the media is hardly classed as a caring profession, and most of our friends came from that world, the warmth and sensitivity shown to both of us was tremendous.

At first people were careful to stay no more than a few minutes because Kim flagged so easily. Before he was able to talk very much they were quite happy to keep up a one-sided conversation. Everything was done with humour and most people made great efforts not to talk down to him; but, above all, whatever they privately felt, they always talked as if it was a matter of *when* Kim got better not *if*. The atmosphere was so positive I knew it must be doing him good.

Most people were terribly shocked when they first saw him and did not believe there could ever be a total recovery, but Kim's weekly improvement was such that those who could bring themselves to make a second visit could feel hope.

One of the reasons for the initial shock was that very few people have any idea of the effects of a serious injury or the results of brain damage. Journalists may feel themselves hardened because of the tragic stories they often have to cover, but it does not prepare them for dealing with personal tragedy. With the professional detachment removed, they were as vulnerable as anybody: this was not some story to be forgotten after transmission or raw material for tales in the pub, this was Kim. It was different.

Even Debbie, a friend who had been a nurse in an intensive care unit, found to her surprise that seeing Kim on a ventilator was terribly upsetting because this was not just another patient, it was somebody she knew.

For the hospital staff, of course, Kim was just part of their job. Months later Dr Oolu, the anaesthetist, came to our house to celebrate Kim's birthday. As we watched Kim talking and laughing to other people he told me this was the first time he had seen Kim as a person; while he was in hospital he was just a body, someone he practised his craft on. And this was the man who had been dragged out of bed at four in the morning to take Kim off the ventilator, and had battled to get Kim breathing again.

The other reason people were shocked at the sight of him was my fault. I was so busy looking on the bright side of Kim's recovery that I painted an extremely rosy picture to other people: I saw him only in terms of his progress. To me he was not a depressing semi-cabbage or someone to be pitied because he was sad and pathetic and not like he used to be; he was getting better, making the most remarkable progress in coping with and overcoming his disability. Kim as he was before the accident had begun to fade into an unreal memory and while I still did hanker for a 'normal' relationship, there was a very deep affection if not love for the person who Kim now was. He was utterly vulnerable, with all the social props which had been built up over his life removed from him, yet he was still coping and just showing what a tremendously nice person he was.

Another reason for my rosy reports was my terror that people would write him off, and this was not for his sake alone. I needed people to see him through my eyes, to see the potential rather than what was missing, so as to reinforce my optimism rather than question it. My worst excess of this was probably with Don Horrabim, who was then Deputy Editor of ITN.

A few days after his parents' visit Kim was having his physiotherapy session in the gym when Don arrived, so I chatted to him while he waited. I had met him once before, in rather happier circumstances, as I waited for the plane carrying Kim back from the Falklands after the war to arrive at RAF Lyneham in Wiltshire. He and an ITN reception committee were waiting for 'their boy' Michael Nicholson. I had not wanted anyone from ITN management to see Kim while he was still unable to hold a conversation, still muddled about everything, with his one wall eye making him appear even more like a dolt, emaciated and walking with a limp, unrecognisable as the young reporter Don knew. How could Don see him and see an ITN reporter? Nobody would believe he could ever return to work.

Instead of doing the sensible thing and warning him that Kim was in a terrible state and seeing him might be rather a shock, though adding that the prospects for recovery were good, I panicked. I painted a glowing picture. Nothing I said was untrue, but all I talked about was the progress and the improvements: how hard he was working at getting better and the admiration of the nursing staff at his efforts.

It was about three-quarters of an hour before Kim eventually returned to the ward. He had been to see the psychologist on the way back from the gym so I knew he would be absolutely exhausted with the physical and mental effort the two visits would have cost him. The odds were against getting one sensible word out of him at all. As he was helped into the ward by a porter I could see him drooping with tiredness. He was not even going to know who Don was.

I gritted my teeth. When he came to his bed I said cheerily: "Kim, look, Don's come to see you. You remember Don Horrabim from ITN don't you?"

Kim took his cue, smiled, nodded and held out his hand.

He sat down in the armchair beside the bed and for the first time held a conversation. He did not just answer Don's questions in sentences, but also asked a few broad questions himself, nothing which would commit himself to knowing to whom he was speaking, but polite queries that were entirely appropriate. He even slung in the odd jokey remark.

As Kim began to flag, Don said he did not want to tire him out and politely said goodbye. In spite of Kim's remarkable performance my heart sank. It was obvious how shocked Don was, but there was nothing I could do. He had seen the situation and would report back accordingly.

When he had left I told Kim I was terribly sorry about the visit but there had been no way of stopping Don. Kim whispered back: "It's all right. It's my job."

That was the first intimation I had had that he had any idea about his work or who he was. Though it was to be some months before he consciously admitted to being an ITN reporter, his instinct for social survival was unimpaired. The nurses could always tell when one of his bosses came to visit him just by his reaction, even though he would say he did not know who they were.

I heard later that Don did not write Kim off. After the visit he told a colleague that he had been extremely shocked at the condition he had found Kim in, which was worse than he had imagined, but no more than that. And ITN never did give up hope. They not only held open his job for him and paid his salary, which was a gread load off my shoulders, but in practical terms demonstrated the same determination as I did that Kim would return to his old job and perform it as well as ever.

I still find the reaction of the people at ITN amazing. He had only worked with them seven months, yet every day at least one person from there would come to visit him and normally many more. As he improved and became more able to cope with people, groups of them would turn up to spend their lunch hours with him or pop in after work throughout the time he was at Queen's Square.

Duncan was one of Kim's first visitors after he was allowed them; as the only person who completely shared my faith in Kim's eventual recovery his observations were terribly important. This was the first time he had been able to see Kim for himself, up until then he had had to rely on my reports for his optimism. When he came he treated Kim as if there was no problem and told him all about the stories he was working on for *City*

Limits, gave him some sports news and related amusing incidents of the past week. He made it easy by asking few questions. Kim obviously understood and followed what he had been told because when Duncan said goodbye he wished him luck with finding a person he was after to back up one of the stories.

I had gone out of the room during the visit because I thought it would be easier for both of them to be left alone, but I returned in time to hear Duncan saying goodbye, promising to come back and visit him soon and telling him he was not nearly as bad as everybody thought he was.

Those words were meant to be cheering to both of us, but I was mortified. I felt I had probably been patronising Kim, and if I had treated him as an equal, as Duncan did, he would be making much better progress. From then on I made a conscious effort to talk to the Kim I had known, a responsible adult person, rather than be put off by the symptoms of brain damage he was exhibiting. I do not pretend I succeeded, but I tried.

The Waldorfs also visited that first weekend. Stephen Waldorf's father, Len, is a freelance cameraman with ITN and he had kept Kim supplied with information during Stephen's subsequent recovery and ensured he was the first to know about any developments. Quite a close relationship developed between the Waldorf parents and Kim, and to a lesser extent Stephen.

Stephen's mother Beryl had been Kim's first outside visitor, while he was still in a coma, before visiting was allowed. She had been reading the *News of the World* (not, she hastened to add, a paper normally seen in her house, but bought because there was an article about Stephen in it) and on the front page there was a paragraph saying Kim was critically ill after an accident in Greece. She had been so upset she just called a taxi and went straight to the hospital to see for herself.

This second visit had the same style. We were enjoying the sun in the grass square outside the hospital, I was reading the Sunday papers and Kim was lolling in his wheelchair when a voice said, "Hello, Kim."

I turned to see a woman I did not know leaning over Kim's wheelchair, chattering away to him. When she realised I was with him she introduced herself then turned back to him to inform him that after what had happened to Stephen she had never wanted to see another intensive care unit in her life; now look what he had gone and done to himself. She talked of him as if he were her son too.

It was touching to see how much she cared. I knew, from being a reporter myself, how seldom any real rapport is struck with people involved in a story, because of the demands of the news desk. I remembered all too well Kim's difficulties in the Waldorf case, when he was torn between pressure from ITN who at times seemed to expect Len Waldorf to put the needs of *News at Ten* before his son, and his moral obligation to the family. By the end the conflict of loyalties was such that he felt neither side was happy with him. It was good to know that Beryl had appreciated his dilemma.

Len turned up an hour later showing the same concern.

That evening Stephen came to visit. Kim was exhausted but there appeared to be some glimmer of recognition even though he was too tired to respond very much. Stephen talked of the horrors of being on a ventilator and his perpetual plans to escape from hospital. Kim remembers neither Stephen's visit nor his time on the ventilator but he has retained an incredible affinity for Stephen. Kim was furious when the policemen who shot Stephen were acquitted.

In many ways Stephen's injuries and Kim's were completely different, but Stephen still had some useful insights. He remembered being given mental arithmetic problems while he was in hospital, presumably to gauge the damage, and described how devastated he felt when he found he could not do simple sums. The numbers just would not add up in his head. He knew he should be able to do it, he knew it was easy, but it just would not come and he was terrified his brain had stopped working. This was obviously happening to Kim all the time, with everything he tried to do.

Stephen also talked about visitors. He said he had found the intervals between visitors very boring and was always longing for another one to turn up but when he did get visitors he soon found them an imposition because of the effort it took to respond to them; but however much he wished they would go away he was always grateful to them for breaking the monotony and they did stimulate his brain to work and pull him out of his lethargical fog.

Certainly it was through his visitors that Kim became gradually more aware of his surroundings and was forced to deal with his condition. He wanted them to return to ease the monotony, and to get over people's embarrassment he turned everything into a joke. In the early days it was just the odd humorous response, as with his rejoinder to Andrew, or simply facial expressions.

Anna Coote, a friend through the NUJ and my immediate boss at Diverse, met me at the hospital one evening to take me out to dinner. Kim was still unsure about his attitude to visitors but I had hoped her visit would buck him up. Before the accident he had slightly idolised her for having brains, wit, politics and good looks; but at this stage his male hormones or whatever were still not quite back in working order and he obviously regarded rest as preferable to entertaining someone. Knowing she would be the last visitor of the day and that after we left he could have all the sleep he wanted, I started trying to cajole some response from him, and wound up his bed to force him to sit up. As I did so there were muttered insults from him. Anna asked if I bullied him *all* the time, to which he just rolled his eyes in an expression of continual suffering. Anna and I started giggling and Kim, realising he was on to a winner, went on trying to elicit sympathy from Anna for the way I treated him – just as he always had done when he felt I was not exhibiting enough concern about his current ailment.

From then on any friend who came to visit could expect to be met with insults; they were called a pudding or a peasant and had to put up with complaints about the calibre of his visitors. He had great fun playing with people's names, picking out any outlandish handle which came to mind. It was his humorous way of dealing with a terrible problem: although he was beginning to recognise most of the people who came to visit him and know how they fitted into his life, he only knew the names of his family, so he would dub people Horace Bluebottle and other imaginings, designed to make people laugh and cover his failure.

I am not even sure when he finally got my name right, because I became Veronica whenever he felt like annoying me, and any other female name which happened to pass through his mind when I turned up to see him.

One of the odd things about Kim's memory was the different levels on which it came back, encapsulated by his attitude to me. To this day he remembers nothing of our life together before the accident; he believes there was one because I have told him so, but not one incident has come back. Yet, according to the nurses, right from the beginning his responses to me were more marked then to anybody else: he would always be more animated in my presence.

At other times he would automatically respond with information he said he did not have. For instance, for months he denied ever having been a television reporter, yet when asked how to do a 'piece to camera' (when the reporter does his little spiel in vision) he explained it easily, even remembering the tricks he used to help him.

That lucidity was in the future; for the moment I was coping with an almost inarticulate man.

Chapter 5

WEEKEND BREAKS

It was now two weeks since Kim had come off the ventilator – a month since the accident. He was able to walk alone and a few sessions in the gym had stopped him dragging his right leg. He was beginning to put on weight and no longer looked dangerously thin, although he was certainly still skinny. His left eye still wandered and the doctors did not know whether the damage to the optic nerve was temporary or permanent.

He could now speak in sentences and would volunteer information without being questioned, but much of what he said did not make sense. A problem with his vocabulary was beginning to show: he could not summon up the correct words on demand. If I held up a comb he would call it a brush, or a clock or a shoe; any noun that occurred to him. This made talking with him difficult because he was often not able to say what he meant. His occupational therapist, Stella Doble, told me the first object he had correctly identified had been a typewriter, and that had been when he was going past one in the occupational therapy department. Clearly his journalism was deeply embedded in his memory bank.

His transposition of words made him appear far more stupid than he was. One day Leslie, the physiotherapist, told me that Kim had been babbling nonsense again: he had been talking about going to the zoo and visiting the white lobster. I told his mother about it on the telephone that night and she said that when Kim was a child one of the great attractions of Bristol Zoo had been a white tiger. He had just muddled his vocabulary again. The scope for misinterpreting him was great even later on, when he was more articulate. He was once asked why he was still speaking in a hoarse voice, long after the sore throat left by the rubbing tubes must have cleared up. He dramatically whispered in reply that his voice had been steamed away. At first I thought he had developed paranoia, but then I remembered the warm, moist oxygen that he had been made to breathe when he was coming off the ventilator. He had hated it at the time, but the nurses had continued to make him breathe it because they were worried he was not getting enough oxygen as his breathing pattern was not yet firmly established.

His speech problems were aggravated by the way his brain damage had affected his memory. His childhood was beginning to come back to him, but most of his life appeared to be a blank and his short-term memory was still crippling: he could only register anything for about five minutes. So he would always deny he had had any visitors, because he could not remember them, and if I went to the loo or to see one of the nurses about something he would greet my return as an arrival, forgetting I had spent the last few hours with him.

There had been a great improvement since he had come off the ventilator but I had been told it was now unlikely that anything was suddenly going to snap back into place. This had been a possibility in the first week off the machine when his medication was reduced, as the muddle could have come from the drugs. Now it was going to be a matter of relearning and slowly bringing his memory back by stimulation. Nobody discussed the possibility of Kim not making a full recovery; the nurses all had stories of people who were much worse and had managed it.

I had to come to terms with the fact that Kim had brain damage, something I had been refusing to admit. My shying away from the term was partly because of the stigma attached to it and partly because of what I thought it meant. To me, brain damage implied people who could not think properly, who were morons, and I knew in Kim's case this was not true. I had always been led to believe that the problems caused by brain damage were irreversible, that once part of the brain was gone, that was the end of whatever function it had, but they were talking about Kim getting better. I discovered that the brain is the most sensitive organ we have, it is easily damaged and takes a very long to heal. If actual cells are destroyed they do not regenerate, but other parts of the brain can compensate for destroyed cells and take over their functions since we make use of only about ten per cent of our brains. In Kim's case the amount of irreversible damage was still unknown because the healing process was only just beginning; like any other part of the body, as his brain got better so the undamaged parts would begin to function properly.

My understanding of all this was not going to lessen the stigma in the outside world. People find brain damage frightening in a way they do not find other physical damage alarming, because it affects the patient's behaviour and they do not understand it. Even I was having difficulty getting over my prejudice about the term and I was dealing with Kim every day knowing reality was different from my misconception of the words.

Those who came to visit often worried about how much time I spent in the hospital because they found it such a depressing atmosphere with so many sad cases in the beds around Kim. In fact I was quite happy there because I felt normal. In the outside world I was an object of pity and sympathy, someone whose suffering set her apart; while on the ward I was just one of the many people whose lives had been ripped apart by illness and accident, and better off than most. I also saw Kim's fellow patients differently: to the others they were hopeless cases with dull eyes and little brain function, but to me they had all become people with individual characters. I was terribly sorry for their relatives but I did not find their condition frightening because I was so used to it. The hospital had become more real for me than life outside; I knew that there lay the seeds of a potentially major problem.

The saddest case was Samer whose parents came from the Lebanon but were living in Britain. He had been in his last year at school when the brain tumour was discovered, so during the long summer holidays between sitting his 'A' levels and taking up his place at University College London he had agreed to have it operated on. Something went wrong after the operation; pressure built up inside the head and he went into a coma. That had been nearly a year ago. Now he was no longer in a coma, but it made little difference. He could open his eyes to see out of them, work his mouth to eat and make bellowing sounds, but that was the limit of his abilities and consciousness. He had originally been in the Italian Hospital, a private institution round the corner from the National, but as the medical bills mounted up he was transferred to NHS care. To the outside world he appeared a hopeless case, but his parents refused to give up. Every morning they would come into the ward and set themselves up on either side of his bed for the day, and they would virtually take over his care from the nurses. His mother would have spent the evening before cooking tempting delicacies for him to eat. She would hug him and try to cajole him into speaking to her, shake him and sometimes gently slap his face in an attempt to provoke a response. During the day his brothers often visited and occasionally even a former school friend. His mother told me there had been some improvement over the months, and obviously she was hoping there would be more. Samer was always treated as a person who could hear and understand in spite of his lack of response, so much so that when Kim's bed was next to his I would not have dreamed of coming or going without giving him the common courtesy of saying hello or goodbye.

There was Graham, a man in his fifties who had had brain problems since he was a child. He had been in and out of hospital all his life. This latest visit was because he had fractured his skull falling down stairs and was now having difficulty making a recovery. He could sit up but not walk and had to be fed through a tube. He probably understood everything that was said to him, but he rarely responded. His wife was becoming quite desperate because she knew he should not be in the ward, which was really only for acute patients, but she could not get him into any rehabilitation centre. He was too old and his prognosis was too doubtful to take up one of the few places. She knew he would not be allowed to keep his valuable bed much longer, and the alternatives were very depressing. The last time he had had trouble he had been put in a geriatric home, where he was tied to a chair and banished to the linen room to stop him being a nuisance. She dreaded him just being written off. Every afternoon she would travel in from the North London suburb where she lived and sit with him, talking about the past, showing him pictures of holidays they had been on together in happier times, or attempt to evoke childhood memories: always trying to provoke a response, desperately attempting to prove there was hope.

Desmond was admitted after Kim had come off the ventilator, for an operation on a brain tumour. During surgery it was found to be larger than at first thought and parts of his brain used for speech were damaged. When he came round from the anaesthetic he found himself semi-paralysed on one side and unable to talk. His intellectual faculties were not affected at all, but his inability to communicate made him appear stupid. He was well aware of this and not only had to develop a new system of communication, he also had to contend with the terrible waves of depression at his impotence. His wife suddenly found their relationship of twenty-odd years turned on its head, and in the beginning blamed herself for not being able to understand his desperate attempts to make his meaning clear. He was not one to bow down to adversity; he laughed as often as he cried, had one of the dirtiest cackles I have ever heard and flirted outrageously with me and all the nurses. He was a forceful man, obviously used to doing everything his own way; he had built up a financially successful life on his own terms and the sudden change in circumstances must have been terrible for him. Although he could no longer talk, occasionally, late in the evening when the ward lights were off, he could be heard quietly singing to himself. I do not know if he was only able to do it in certain circumstances or just refused to be treated like a performing monkey, but he never did it during the day and so I never heard him.

When I was back at work Kim was in a bed next to Desmond. They had a wonderful relationship. Desmond would patiently watch Kim's antics and listen to his constant repetitions, then when I came to visit and asked Kim about his day Desmond would nod in agreement or shake his head to correct Kim's many wrong answers. When Kim swore blind that nobody had visited him, as he did every day, Desmond would pat me on the hand and shake his head to reassure me Kim had not been left in solitude.

I forget quite what was the matter with Mario, but whatever it was, by the time Kim was admitted he was getting better, though not making the dramatic sort of improvements Kim made. Mario mostly sat slumped in a chair, and it was difficult to talk to him because he was Maltese and spoke no English. This communication problem made him appear worse than he was. Regular visits from his brother stopped him from feeling totally isolated in the ward.

Jonathan was about seventeen. He had had a tumour on his spine since the age of nine, so he was confined to a wheelchair. He had come up from his home in Cornwall for tests because he had sores on his back from the constant rubbing. They had been left untreated for so long that his condition had become serious and he had been told he would have to be transferred to the orthopaedic hospital at Wembley in North London and stay there for nine months while skin grafts were done. His parents were not going to be able to afford to stay in London all that time, so Jonathan, with all his friends in Cornwall, would spend most of the time alone. I spoke to him most days, and liked him a lot. He spent much of the time doing beautifully intricate drawings, and although he was unhappy at the prospect of another nine months in hospital, somehow he was not overcome by depression.

Then there was Eamon, the mugging victim who had been admitted during Kim's last relapse. His condition was far more serious than Kim's had been and his family were warned there was little hope. Once they spent the whole night around his bed because they had been told he probably would not see the morning. Later his ventilator was switched off to see if there would be any reaction and incredibly he started breathing alone. I began to think miracles were commonplace on the ward. As soon as he was stable he was transferred to a hospital nearer his family, so I could not follow his progress and compare it to Kim's, but he was alive, which was more than anyone had thought possible at first. The staff in the hospital at Queen's Square would fight for anyone's life, however hopeless it seemed, until there was no life left.

The ward did not depress me but I was worried about its effect on Kim. He always refused to talk about where he was. I was convinced he thought himself in a mental hospital. His mind was alert enough to be working things out, and likely as not coming to the wrong conclusion. I decided Kim needed a visit home, it would give him some hope and get him out of the ward. It was a terrible problem trying to explain to Kim what was wrong with him: a person with a broken leg cannot walk but understands the problem, but Kim's very faculties for understanding and communication were affected. Like Desmond he not only had to overcome and cope with the problems brought on by brain damage, but I felt he also found the effects of what had happened to him so frightening he was not sure he wanted to know what it was. I thought that back at home it would perhaps be easier to explain, and in familiar surroundings it might be easier for him to understand and see there was hope for him. I also believed that merely getting him out of an institution and back into some semblance of normal life would help; perhaps it would jog something and things would fall into place.

Kim also wanted to go home, although I am not sure he truly knew what it was. Once when we were doing our circuits of the ward he stopped beside Sister Thorman, jerked his thumb at me and said, "I want to go away with her." As courtship went it was rather crude, but it was nice to know he cared. Sister Thorman explained to him that it would be a while before he could come home with me for good, but soon he would be allowed out for a weekend.

Kim now had few medical problems so I decided the time had come. Mr Hayward gave his permission and Friday, 10 June, the day after the general election, was D-Day.

A couple of days before he was due to come home Sister Kennedy asked me to have tea with her in her office. She had known someone well who had been in a similar accident to Kim's and talked a lot about what had happened to him.

She said, "The first weekend is very funny, you laugh a lot." She paused and looked at me. "You have to laugh. . .or else you would cry."

But I was too excited to take much notice.

I had been wondering whether Kim should vote at the election. I was sure the hospital would allow me to drive him to his polling station; it would require quite a lot of organisation but it was certainly possible. In the end I decided not to bother, partly because it was easier, but mostly because I was not sure he had all his political faculties back. He had been a member of the Labour Party since he was eighteen and Mrs Thatcher's first term in office had certainly done nothing to weaken his allegiance; but now when I asked him who he would vote for he would only say Mrs Thatcher. I knew he would never forgive me if I allowed him to vote Conservative, but it seemed to be cheating to make him put a cross where I told him rather than choose himself, so I decided not to try.

He still refuses to believe he really could ever have said good things about her. When I tease him about it he mutters, "I MUST have been barmy."

I watched the election results with Duncan and Julie Christie at the house of people who worked with Duncan at *City Limits*, John Fordham and Ros Asquith. It was depressing watching the Tories sweep the board. The only two bright spots were that Duncan's canvassing had not been in vain, Jeremy Corbyn had ousted the SDP man in Islington North, and in the Montgomery constituency where Julie lived in her Welsh farmhouse, the hard-line Tory lost his seat to a Liberal. Ros and I were the only ones naive enough to believe Labour had any hope – I just could not understand how people could vote Conversative – the others were resigned to a defeat.

As dawn broke I drove Duncan and Julie home, dropping them at the end of Duncan's street. Julie was wearing a beautiful circular skirt and Duncan was dressed in a slightly fifties style himself, and I sat and watched them skip through the slight mist which heralded the heat of the coming day: they were like two teenagers from another era.

I went to bed and woke a few hours later feeling depressed at the election results, elated about Kim coming home and exhausted from lack of sleep. Stupidly I thought I would be able to catch up by going to bed early that night.

On the way to the hospital I went to Safeways supermarket and bought boxes of enticing food for the weekend, to tempt Kim's appetite. My supreme sacrifice was to buy a joint of lamb and sausages and bacon so he could have a traditional meat and two veg supper and his favourite big fry-up for breakfast. I do not eat meat and in the past had always refused to cook the bits of dead animals he had brought into the house, but I would do almost anything to build him up again.

When I went to the hospital there was an air of despondency on the ward: a Conservative victory was disastrous news for the Health Service. The nurses knew their conditions would get worse and we visitors knew there was going to be more pressure on rehabilitation places as the cuts went on biting, which meant less chance of decent care once the patients had left the ward, less likelihood of a full recovery or, in some cases, a halt to any potential progress.

Kate Holman, whose boyfriend Aidan I had embarrassed when I was on tranquillisers, had offered to come and stay with me for a fortnight to help and she came to the hospital that afternoon to assist me in getting Kim home. I packed his clothes, was given his pills for the weekend and suddenly we were outside hailing a taxi and on our way home.

During the drive home Kim seemed pleased to be out of the hospital, but he could have been in any city in the world, he recognised nothing. He did not know the house and even indoors everything appeared to be strange to him. I told him this was home and wondered what the word meant to him.

I had set up a bed downstairs in the sitting-room so Kim could sleep whenever he wanted, without having to go all the way upstairs to our bedroom at the top of the house for his naps. It also meant I could keep an eye on him in case he started wandering around the house; he was so disoriented he did not know where anything was.

The greatest problem was the loo. He could not remember where it was and was still so embarrassed about asking that he would never make it plain what he wanted and still asked to go for a walk. This was hardly a practical euphemism since quite often he really did want to go for a walk – it was weeks before he could sit down for more than a few minutes without jumping up to take a turn round the room, house or garden. When he was at home a few weekends later he plaintively announced he wanted to go for a walk just as I was trying to get up the energy to go and buy a bottle of wine for people coming over that evening. I did not even consider the alternative meaning, I just told him he could accompany me to the off-licence. Halfway there he told me he had not wanted to go for a walk at all, but needed a piss. I burst out laughing and told him this was what happened if he insisted on behaving so coyly. He would have to start making his requests more plainly, then we would not have these misunderstandings. To underline my point we went on to the off-licence (a mere hundred yards) and bought the wine before returning home and letting him relieve himself. There were no more euphemisms after that and he even began finding the loo on his own.

That first evening at home he mostly ate and slept. Supper was rather long and drawn out because he had to take a nap between every course, but he proved that given reasonable food he had not lost his appetite. Nevertheless I found the evening exhausting because when he was not eating or sleeping he was impossible to keep occupied for any length of time. He could not concentrate on anything, and would even get up from the table to walk around the room when he got bored of sitting down. It was difficult to talk to him for more than a few minutes and if he was not wandering about he would be fidgeting in his chair, constantly trying to find a comfortable position. He could not watch television because he could not concentrate and his wandering eye did not allow him to focus. My problems were magnified by my exhaustion from the lack of sleep the night before. So we went to bed early.

For the first time I felt slightly frightened at being with Kim. Lying in our bed naked and alone with him I felt very vulnerable; if he turned violent he could strangle me in seconds. It sounds melodramatic, and I now know it was just my overactive imagination mixing too many half-memories of uninformed opinion and prejudice about the effects of brain damage, but I thought that lying there with no clothes on, touching in bed, could cause deep sexual stirrings which might bring out a violent streak in him. I reassured myself with the thought that he would not have been allowed home if there had been any danger of that. At the same time it felt extremely good to be once again lying in bed with Kim; he was so skinny he was a bit bony to be next to, but it was nice to be cuddled again after so long. Far from his deepest feelings being provoked, all he wanted to do was go to sleep.

Unfortunately not for long.

He woke up hourly, always wanting to go to the loo. The first few times I directed him down to it, then sat on the stairs waiting for him to finish so I could bring him back to bed with me. Once I felt so exhausted I went back to bed after showing him the way down, telling myself he would be able to find his own way back. A quarter of an hour later I awoke with a jolt, alone and went downstairs to find Kim wandering around, lost and unhappy.

At about seven he decided it was time to get up and he told me he wanted to get dressed. Through a blur of exhaustion I pointed to the clothes and told him if he wanted to get up that was fine.

I was awoken a few minutes later by the sound of cloth tearing. I opened my eyes to see him struggling to get into a cotton top of mine, ripping it as he forced it over his massive shoulders. I gave an anguished cry and told him it was mine and he had spoilt it. He just started abusing it as though it had done something wrong. Between us we eventually managed to get it off him. I then noticed he had layers and layers of clothes on: tiny T-shirts of mine pulled tight over shirts and jumpers belonging to him. On his bottom half he had on two pairs of shorts and a couple of pairs of trousers half pulled up. He had no idea of the purpose of various types of clothing.

I persuaded Kim to dress himself conventionally and took him downstairs to give him something to drink. Kate was already up and when she noticed I was barely functioning through tiredness she shooed me back upstairs to get some more sleep while she looked after him.

I got up a couple of hours later when Kate went out, and Kim and I spent most of the rest of the day alone. I found it hard work, not only waiting on his every need but also trying to communicate with him. Much of the time he was content to be quiet, and although I felt guilty about not providing much stimulation I let it be that way: just leaving the hospital and coming home provided enough new experiences. But the novelty had caused him to regress; the difficulty of coping with the unfamiliarity made him less coherent. It was a strain, with no nurses or visitors for distraction, but it did mean we became closer and over that weekend I began to develop ways of understanding him. Whenever he appeared to want something I would run through a list of options and he would stop me when I reached the correct one. He still lacked initiative but would respond to suggestions. Mostly he wanted to eat, drink, sleep or go to the loo, so it was quite easy.

Kate came back in the evening and the three of us spent it together. It was better than the previous one, but still hard work keeping up a semblance of conversation. Kim must have sensed the atmosphere because fairly late in the evening he suddenly rounded on me and told me I should leave him and go off with someone else. He rambled on incoherently for a while, sounding quite angry. I felt he knew what a strain I was finding the weekend and was trying to do the honourable thing by offering me my freedom, though he could just as well have been telling me to bugger off out of his life. Whatever he meant I felt assaulted by his anger. It was the last straw at the end of an exhausting day and I was almost in tears trying to answer him and calm him down. Kate had to take over and placate him.

I took him upstairs to our bedroom and by the time we were undressed and in bed it was easy to deal with the situation quite calmly. I told him I had no intention of leaving him, and was going to stay until he got better. If he wanted to get rid of me then, that was fine. Once again I tried to explain what he had wrong with him and, more importantly, stressed that it was going to get better.

That night was as bad as the previous one. Once when he awoke I felt I just could not pull myself out of bed to take him down the stairs to the loo, so I pragmatically decided he would be able to manage it alone and sank back under the duvet. Minutes later I was awakened by the sound of peeing in the corner. For the rest of the night I diligently accompanied him downstairs.

Kate looked after him in the morning while I tried to catch up on some sleep; but Kim started missing me, so he climbed the stairs to our room, then lay down beside me, which was his attempt to let me go on sleeping. But his disturbance combined with the heat of the morning in our attic room meant I could not return to my slumbers.

Kate found Kim very difficult to deal with because she was unsure of how to treat him. She had not known him very well before the accident although she had been fond of him. Both of them are fairly reserved people. She diffidently tried to treat him as the Kim she had known, but found him uncontrollable and at times frightening. Whatever inhibitions he had about asking for the lavatory he had none about taking down his trousers whenever he felt like it. He sensed her timidity and it made him extremely unsure of himself. When he went off into an incoherent ramble she would desperately try to understand what he wanted to say, attempting to follow the thread which even he would have lost by then. She told me later she had really hated being left alone with him.

Kim's brother Richard and his wife Fiona came for lunch. I had asked them because of the difficulty Richard had in visiting Kim in hospital after work; he worked at the Oxford University Press in Oxford, and rarely left the office in time to catch Kim before the end of visiting time. The nurses were understanding about him coming later, but by that time of the day Kim was too worn out to respond to him very much. I also thought it would be nice for Kim to see a familiar face. I did not realise how pleasant it would be for me to have two people who were both undemanding and helpful and could share some of the responsibility for Kim.

After lunch there was an international football match on the television with Brazil playing. Kim was not very interested though he would normally have been glued to the set. He stayed for a while with Richard, chatting to him about the match in a desultory fashion, but soon got fed up and started wandering about, then lay down for a nap. None of us realised at the time just how bad his eyes were; trying to make sense of the match with his double vision must have been almost impossible.

Later in the afternoon Amanda came round. Kim had been upstairs having a rest. He had stripped down to his underpants in the heat and came downstairs to greet her wearing only raggedy blue knickers. I sent him upstairs to dress properly and minutes later he reappeared complaining that his shorts no longer fitted him. No wonder. He was wearing one of my T-shirts, with one of his legs through the neck hole and the other stretching an armhole. So I took him upstairs, helped him put on a pair of shorts and demonstrated the correct way to wear a T-shirt, making sure it was one of his.

When I brought him into the sitting-room, properly dressed, Amanda had put on her glasses. She peered at me intently then started laughing. Without them on she had thought my dark rings from sleeplessness were black eyes from being knocked about by someone.

I turned to Kim and said, "Look who's come to visit you. It's Amanda. You remember her, don't you?"

"Yes. Of course I do," he barked. "She's potty, absolutely potty."

Amanda immediately acted extremely hurt and told him he had got the wrong person, but I roared with laughter and told her he obviously had some brains left.

He kept showing Amanda his knee, which had an enormous scab on it – the cut had originally gone so deep it had chipped part of his bone. He was obviously trying to elicit sympathy. For weeks he did this whenever he had visitors at home; when wearing long trousers he would struggle to pull up the trouser leg. I eventually realised he thought people did not know he had had a terrible accident; he could not see how shocking he looked to them, and he was showing them proof of his sufferings to gain their sympathy. Little had changed, he was always going to indulge his every illness.

When I took him back to hospital that evening he seemed quite pleased. One of the nurses asked how he had enjoyed himself and he said he had had a boring time. I did not have the energy to feel hurt.

By the next morning he denied ever having been home.

In spite of his complete ingratitude he started coming home every weekend until he left hospital.

When I got back home I felt exhausted. The weekend had drained me of most of my shallow reserve of strength and energy. I told Kate that I would have to have a break if I was going to be of any use to anyone for much longer. I decided to go and stay in a small hotel some friends of mine had enjoyed a few months earlier on the Suffolk coast. Kate offered to come with me to make it a happy holiday rather than a solitary rest cure.

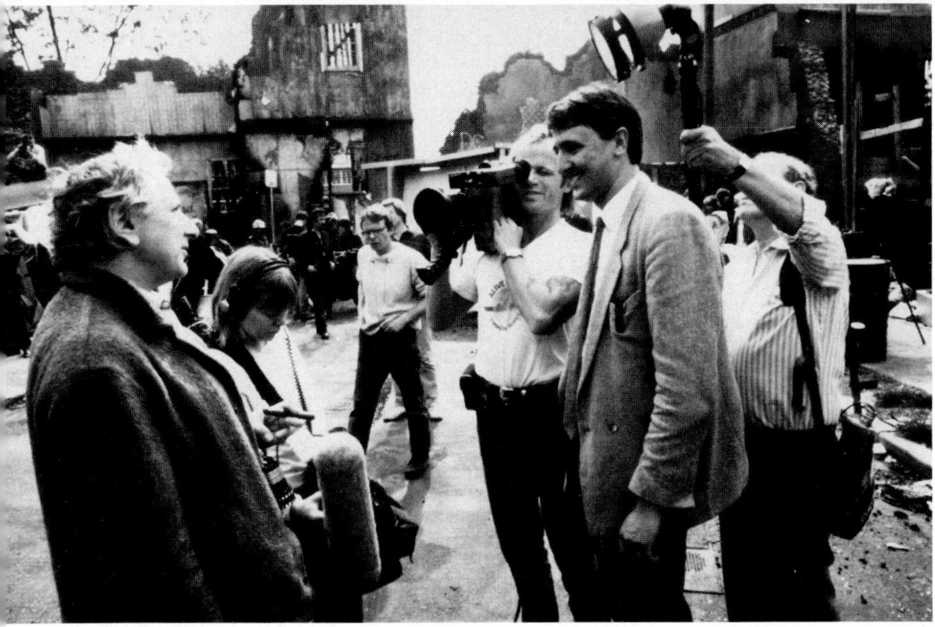

ɔve: Kim on the set of *Death Wish III* in London, interviewing the director, Michael Winner with camera operator, Sebastian Rich

ɔw: Kim in the Falklands for *ITN* in 1983

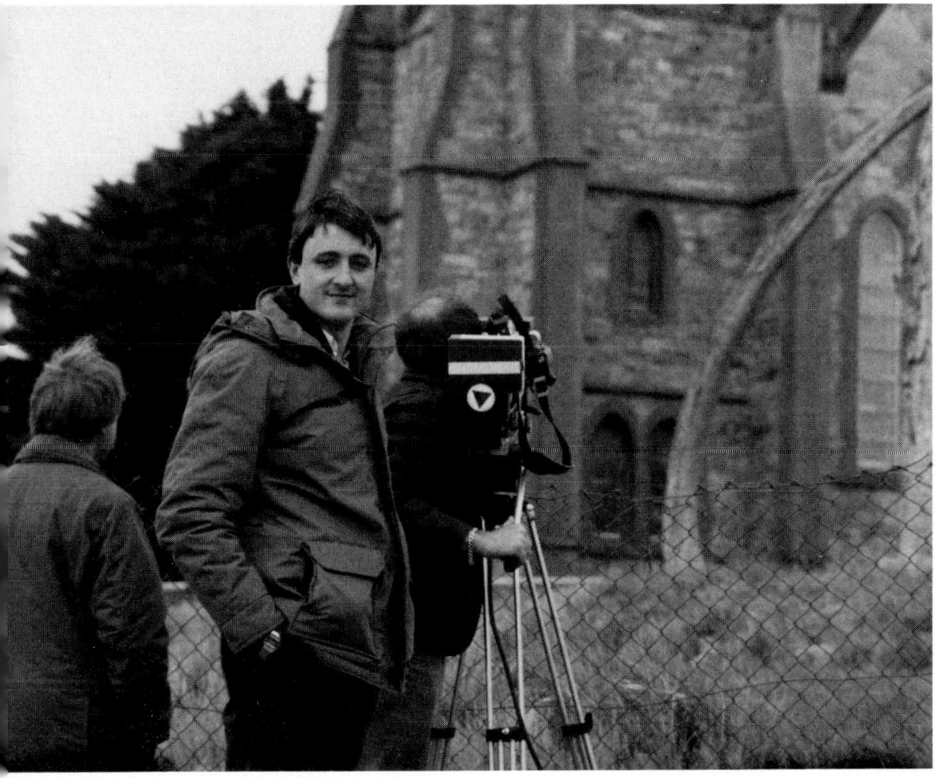

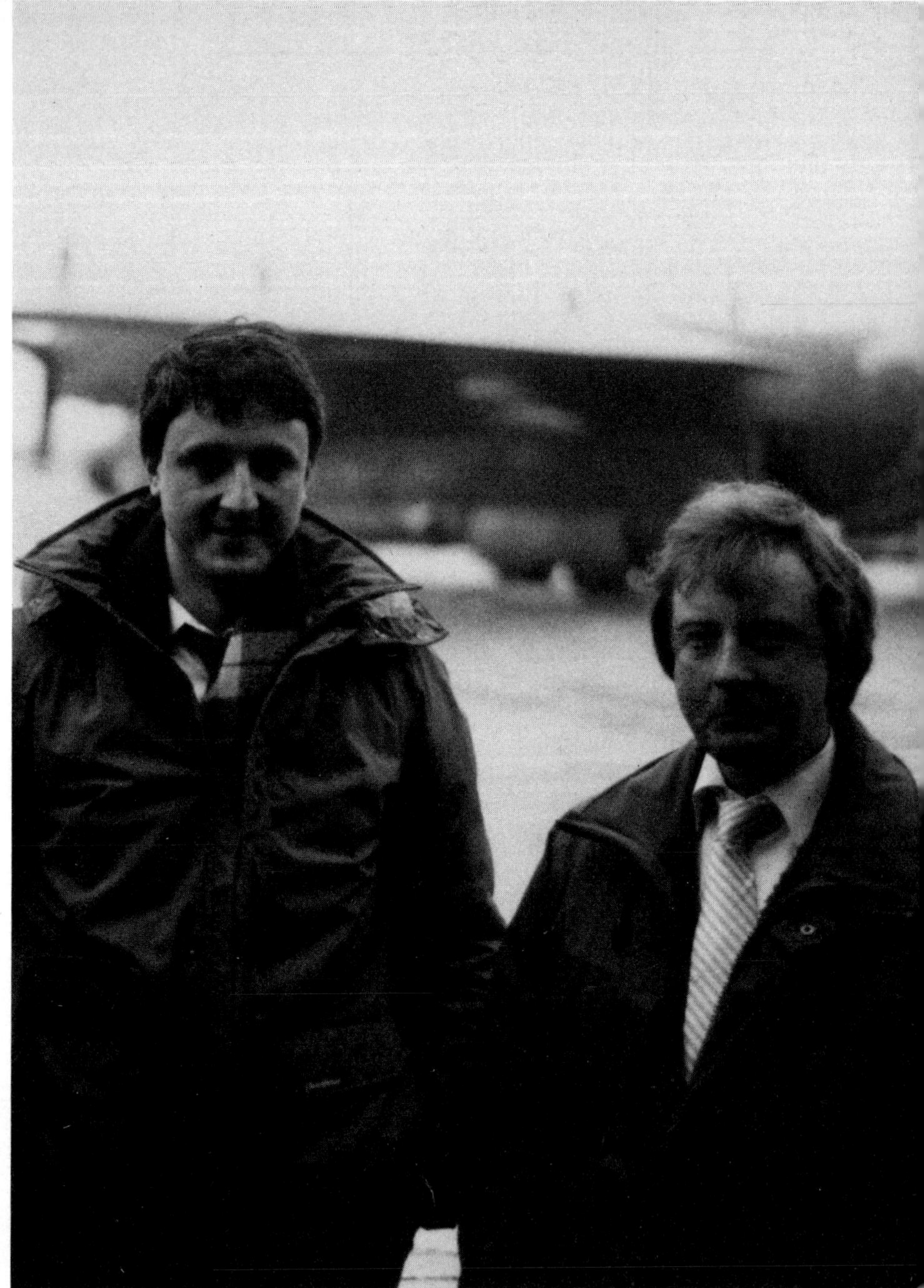

Above: Kim with Nicholas Witchell from the *BBC* in the Falklands

Above Right: Kim's father in the garden at home

Right: Kim's mother with Pascoe at two weeks old

Far Right: Scarlett and her mother at a wedding in 1979

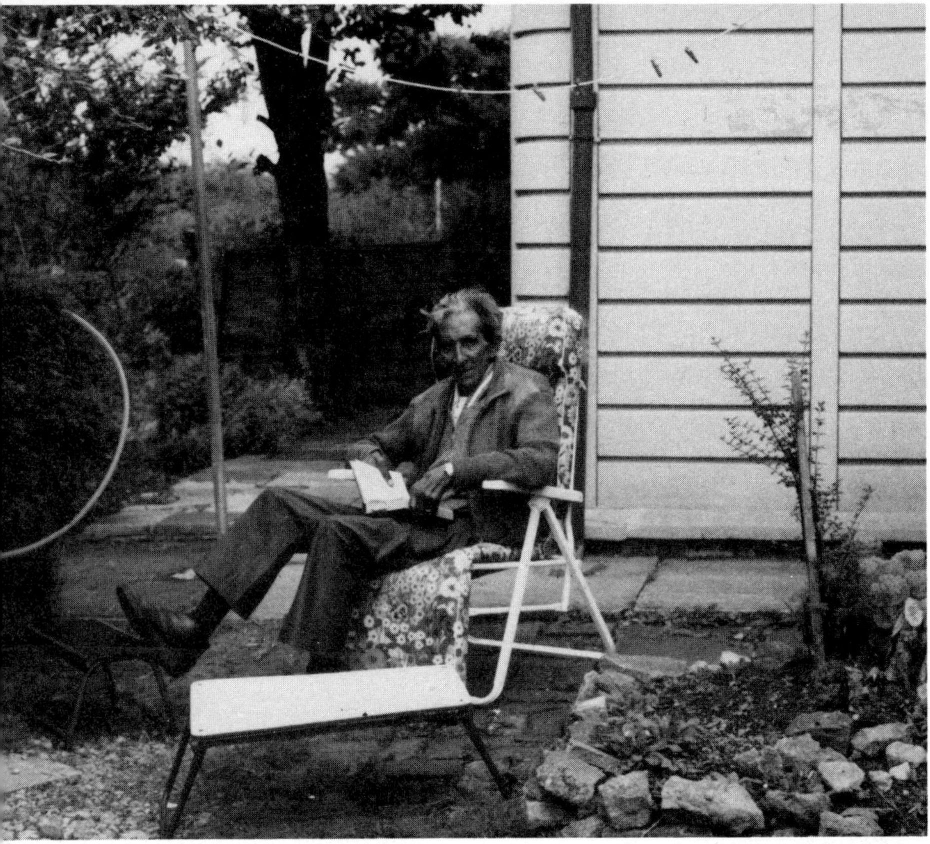

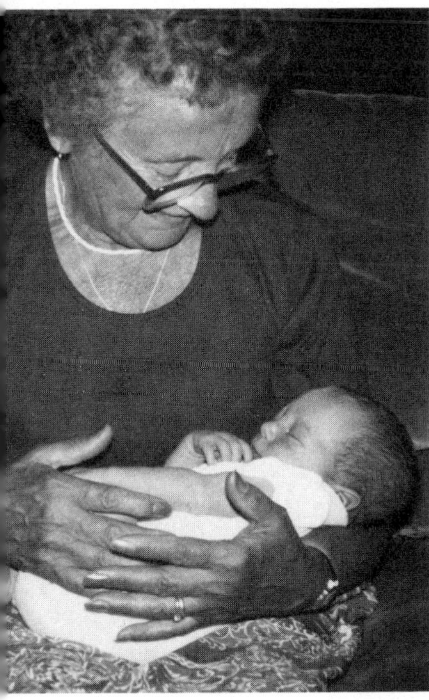

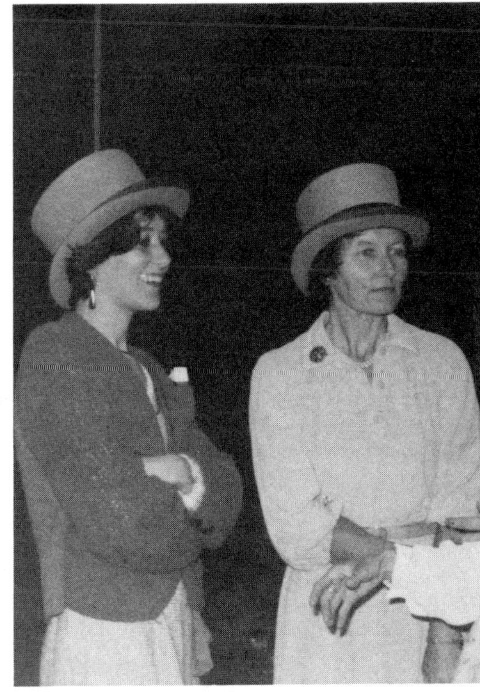

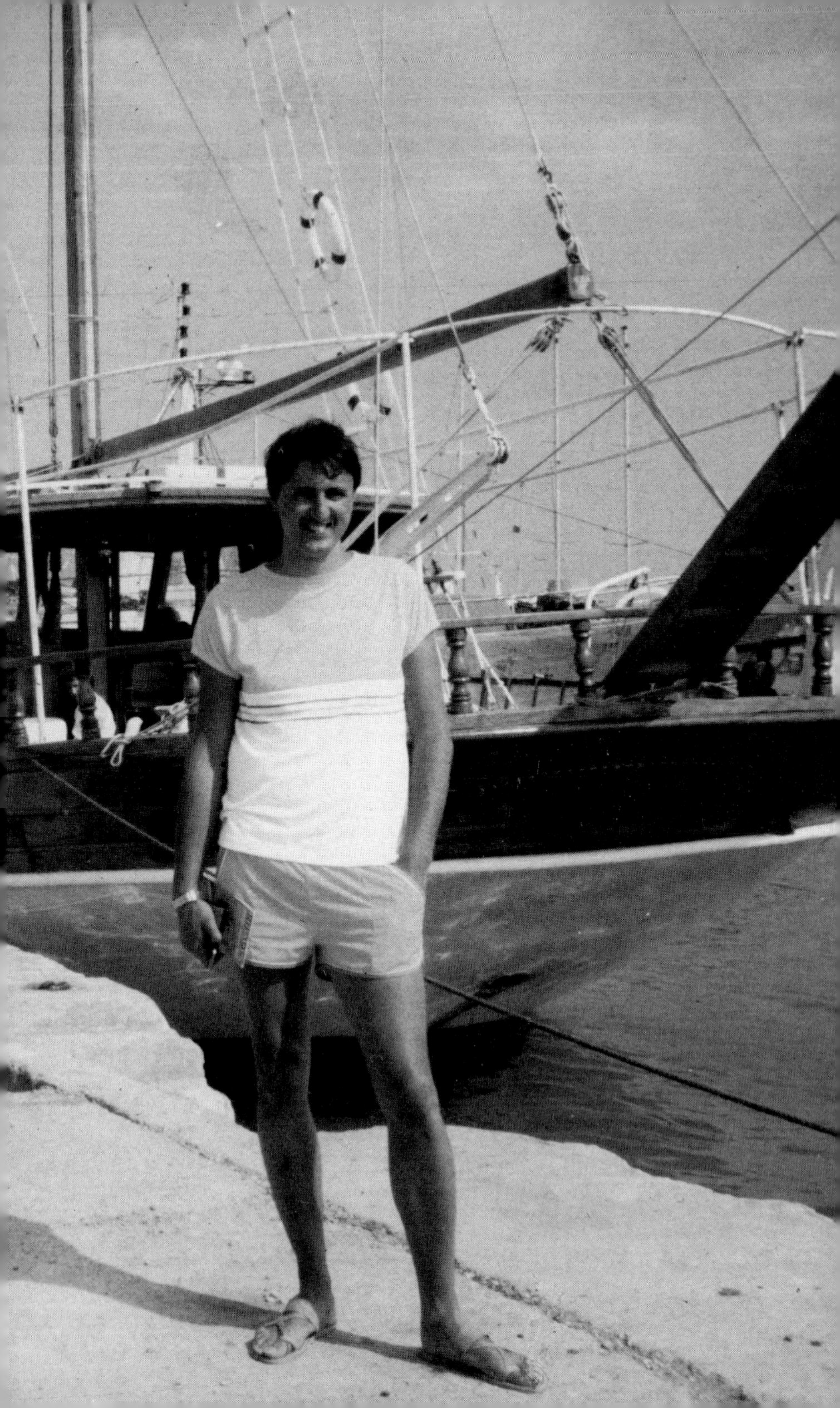

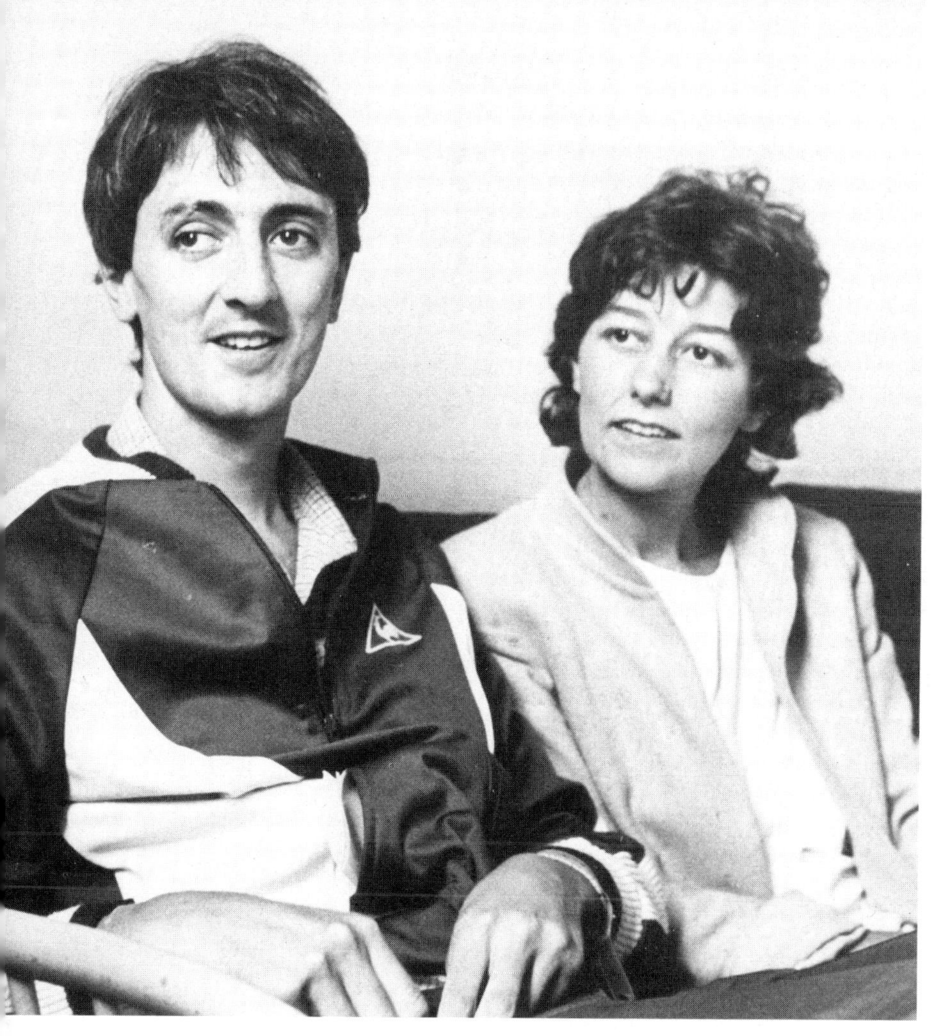

Kim at the harbour in Rhodes Town an hour before the accident

e: Kim and Scarlett six weeks after the accident

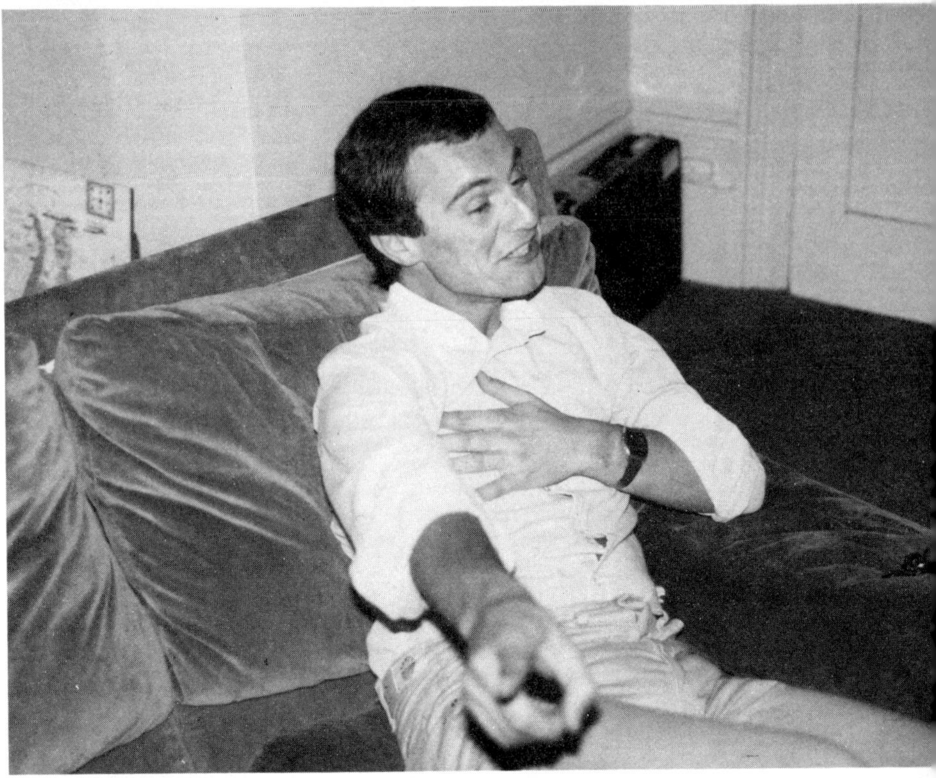

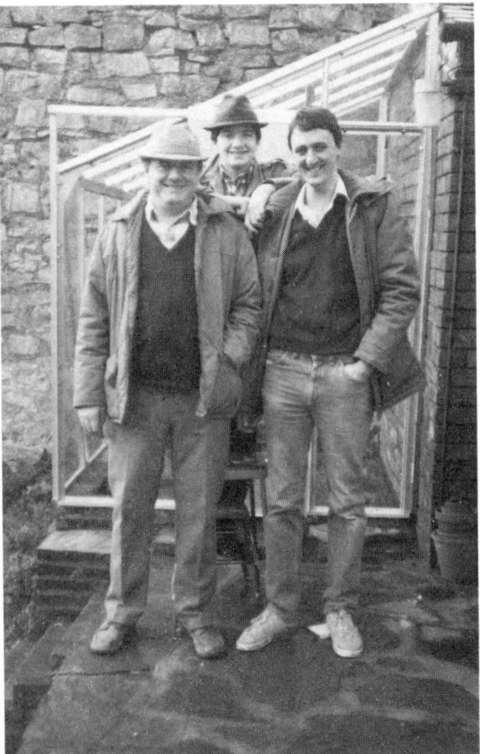

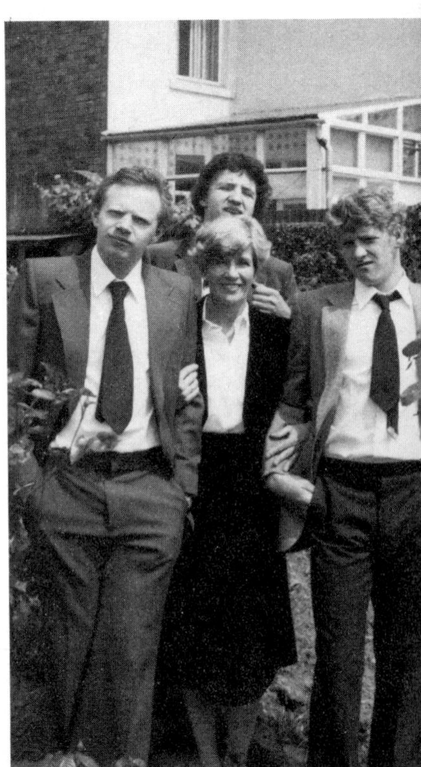

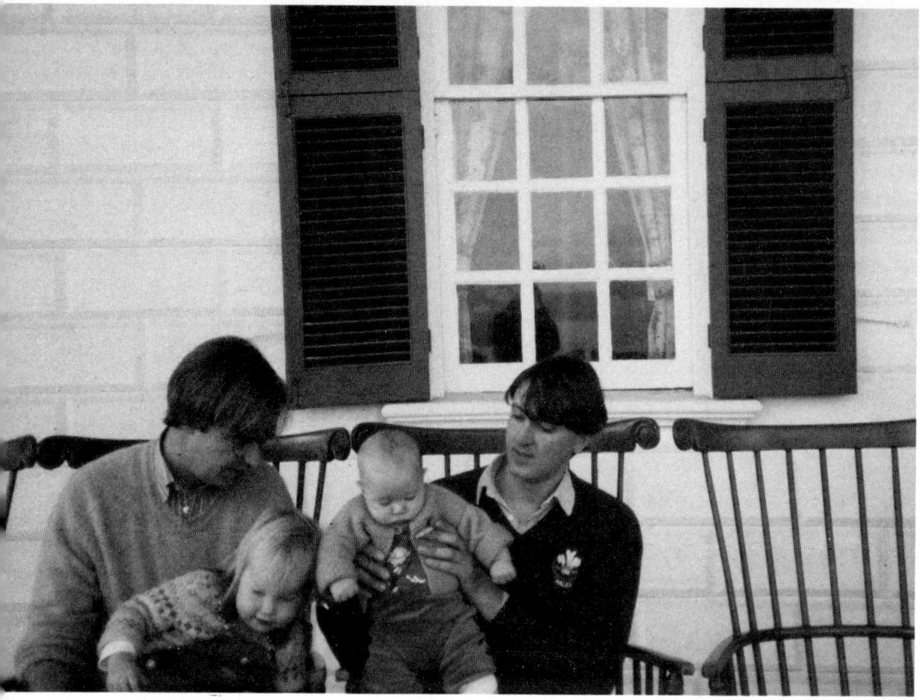

left: John Draper

ft: From left to right, Brian Hurley,
ı Robert and Kim

'at Hurley with her sons *(from left to*
Jonathan, David and Simon Hurley

: Jon Snow and Kim with Leila and
e

Ferdie Dennis in the old *City Limits*
in Islington

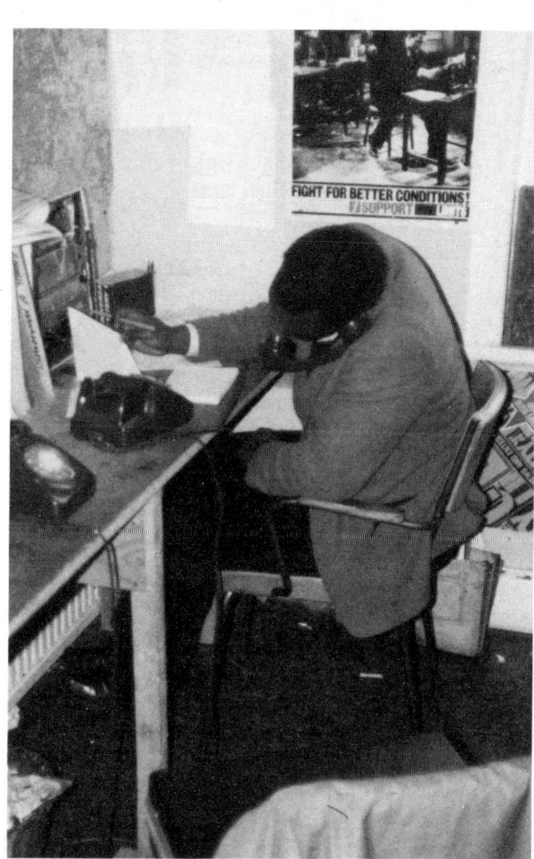

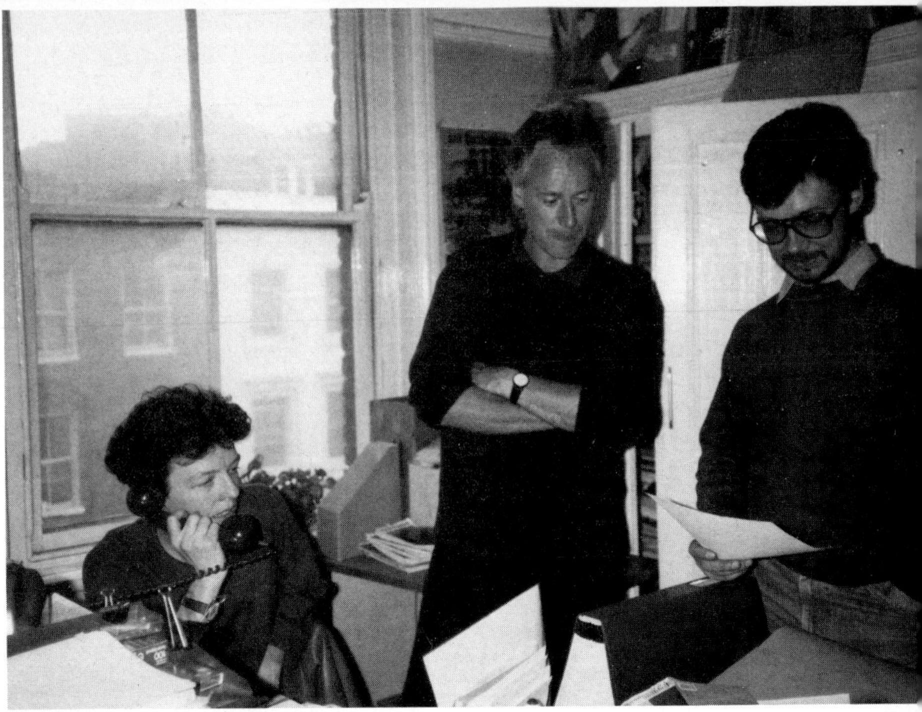

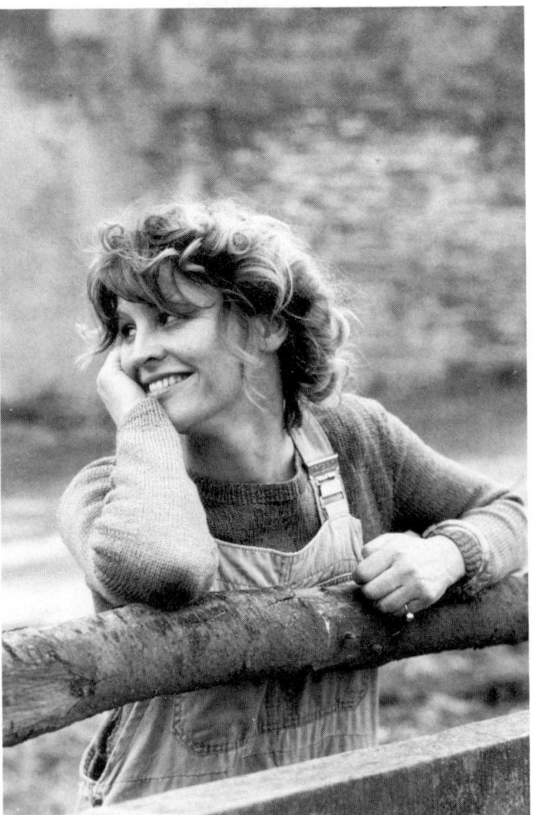

Above: Left to right: Bea Campbell, D
Campbell and Steve Pinder at *City Li*

Left: Julie Christie on her farm in Wa

It was wonderful. We stayed at the King's Head in Alford. The first evening we went to a nearby pub for supper and I got gloriously drunk; with every sip of beer my troubles grew lighter and began to recede into an alcoholic haze. For the first time in weeks I was able to relax. The village was on an estuary, so the next morning we went down to the waterfront to look at the boats and walked for miles along the banks, sometimes talking, sometimes silent, pleasuring in each other's company, breathing in that wonderful air.

Alford was a tourist haunt, but during the week in term time it was empty and we could enjoy it quietly at our leisure, solitary sightseers. It was as if I had entered a time warp. Kim and the hospital seemed to belong to another life, though it was only ten hours since I had seen him. As the holiday was only three days long I spent every minute savouring my freedom from duty, enjoying the fresh sounds and smells, glorying in being normal. To the few people in the village who noticed us we were just temporary refugees from London; they were used to our sort, we excited no interest. Kate and I talked of the past and of ideas, wishes and dreams – both of us needed a break from the present and had our worries about the future. I slept wonderfully and succumbed to my exhaustion, even indulging in afternoon naps. For every meal I was ravenously hungry instead of just pushing food down me because I knew it was necessary. For that short time, life did not revolve around the hospital and I could revel in the normal, trivial pleasures of daily life.

I was only out of London for a total of fifty-six hours, yet that brief interlude gave me the chance to catch my breath and ready myself for the coming months. I now accepted it would be a long hard battle. I greeted every improvement with excitement but I no longer expected immediate results. I had given up hope of an instant miracle. Kate and I promised ourselves that when everything was fine again we would come back with Kim and Aidan, to show them where we had run away to. Part of me had begun to doubt that that day would ever come. Being with Kim so much made it difficult to believe there could be such an improvement that everything could return to normal again; but I told myself these thoughts were counterproductive, I had to believe in his recovery to make him believe it too.

I visited him the evening we returned to London and found he had missed me. That awareness was progress in itself. He had had a stream of visitors, so it was not loneliness; it showed he had some idea who I was. I had told the nurses of my planned holiday before I went away, and they had encouraged me to take the break, knowing how much I needed it. I had also told Kim about it the day before I went, over and over again, assuring him that I would be back and saying I was not trying to get away from him, but going just to get some rest. He had remained convinced I had had enough of him, and kept telling the nurses I was not coming back. They told me he had become quite doleful. I felt slightly guilty about making him feel unhappy, but knowing how much good the separation had done me I felt he would gain from it in the end.

The second weekend home was much easier than the first. I got a proper night's sleep on the Thursday, leaving me ready for anything Kim had in store for me; I had lower expectations and Kim was not so bemused. While he still did not quite regard it as home he made it plain he liked the change from hospital.

On the Saturday John Draper came to see him. John had worked with us both at LBC/IRN where he was a reporter. He was a Northern Ireland Protestant and he and Kim had always kept up a jokey feud between the Protestant and Catholic; with me he just pretended to be an old reactionary, always provoking arguments. He was very important to us because he was the only close friend we had who was really a friend of both of us; we had both known him before we got together.

John and Kim went for a stroll round our small garden where they had a fairly coherent conversation interspersed with only a few ramblings. As they were coming inside, Kim turned to John and said, "Don't take any notice of anything I say, it's all nonsense."

John found this quite upsetting because so much of what Kim had been saying had made perfect sense; Kim was beginning to use self-deprecation as a defence against anybody thinking that he was not aware of his problems.

John stayed for supper and dubbed Kim 'Two Dinners Sabido', after *Private Eye*'s nickname for Lord Goodman. The allusion was quite justified. Kim wolfed down enormous second helpings of everything, eating twice as much as either of us. John cheered us both up and made me feel less like a social pariah: I felt nobody could possibly choose to spend a Saturday night with us when they could be out having fun. As he always had done in the past, John was rude to Kim and argued with me, so all three of us enjoyed the evening. During the next few months we were to spend many Saturday nights like that. John never realised how important those evenings were, but the three of us, sitting around joking, made everything appear much more manageable. And it made Kim happy, which was the primary reason for his coming home at the weekends.

The suppers also gradually made Kim behave in a socially acceptable manner. At first when he was tired during a meal he would lie his head down next to the plate and I would have to cajole him into going to lie on his bed in the corner. He would finish his course when he woke up about twenty minutes later. John never appeared phased by this, just made some sarcastic remark about the manners of his host. But gradually Kim made an effort to keep awake for the whole meal and have his sleep afterwards, quite often going upstairs for the night as soon as we had finished supper.

On the Sunday of that second weekend, Kate brought round a Welsh friend of hers. I hoped Dai's accent might bring back some memories to the nationalistic Kim, and also wondered whether Kim could still speak or understand Welsh. Dai spoke to him in Welsh and Kim haltingly replied, occasionally breaking into English. Considering the difficulty he had expressing himself in his mother tongue, to understand and even make a stab at speaking a second language, only learned when he was eighteen, was a great achievement. We then tested him in French which again he could understand, though he had more difficulty finding the words to construct a proper reply.

The third weekend Kim's parents were staying with his brother Richard in Amersham, so on the Saturday we went over there for lunch and tea. Earlier that morning my sister Katrina had come round to see Kim, and had looked after him for a while so I could so some shopping. When I returned she said he had been fine, but she had experienced some difficulty understanding him. He had taken to his bed with exhaustion and had asked her to put a cover on his feet, which she found perplexing because he already had a blanket over them; eventually he made it plain that he was actually asking for a pillow for his head.

I had begun to work out ways of overcoming his continual transposing of words. If possible I would make him point to what he was talking about so that when he came to me complaining about his feet hurting I would ask him to point to his feet, and when he pointed to his eyes I would understand what the problem was. His eyes frequently bothered him and there was little I could do except to tell him to sit away from sunlight for a while and regularly remind the nurses that his eyes were giving him trouble. I was always told that in time his left eye might correct itself and he would be able to focus again.

When I told Kim we had to leave for Amersham and Katrina had to go home, he became very upset. First of all he did not want to leave and then he tried to persuade Katrina to come with us as he did not want to part from her. He refused to be satisfied with assurances that she would visit again, but eventually I persuaded him to get in the car and we were off.

His parents were delighted by the improvement Kim showed out of hospital. They had visited Queen's Square the day before and his father had found Kim's happy acceptance of his condition extremely depressing: he would meekly smile at any jokes, do whatever he was asked and mostly try to be a model patient. His father was worried that Kim was not trying to fight his disabilities. But relaxing in Richard's large back garden and playing ball with his nephews and niece, Kim was far more sparky. He also had a visit from a special friend, a marine whom he had met in the Falklands, Cameron March. To jog his memory Richard played Kim a tape of one of his despatches during the Falklands war which mentioned Cam, he and Kim sat apart so he would have Kim's complete attention and stand a better chance of having a sensible conversation; whatever was said between them, Cam appeared satisfied when he left.

When I told Kim we had to get ready to go home because a friend of his was coming down from Scotland to see him and staying the night, he started making a fuss. His parents felt I was dragging him away unwillingly and his father told me I should have not made the arrangement with David. I did not tell them he had made exactly the same fuss earlier when we had left my sister, and she was a person he had only met a few times and did not even remember. He was just afraid of leaving people because he did not want to be left alone. But his father was right about the evening arrangement, because the exertions of the day had worn Kim out. That did not change the time I wanted to leave, however, as I had to drive Kim back to London – we had agreed he was not ready to stay in another house as it would have been too confusing – and I did not want to drive back exhausted in the dark, with Kim possibly deciding he was bored of the journey and insisting we stop, or trying to get out. When I had planned the day I was not sure Kim would be able to stay in the car for the hour's drive, because he had never managed to sit still that long before.

When we finally arrived home David was pleased to see Kim – he had not seen him since before the accident – but it took only minutes for him to realise Kim's condition was far more serious than I had led him to believe; I had talked only in terms of his progress, not properly preparing him for the shock of meeting this completely changed person.

They had met when they worked together on Swansea Sound, David a trainee and Kim a senior journalist. Together with Ian Parkinson (now on Radio One's *Newsbeat*), they made a terrible trio. David had gone on to Kim's old stomping ground, Radio Forth in Edinburgh. Their tales of life at Radio Froth, as they both referred to it, were hilarious. Like most commercial radio stations it appeared to be held together by paper clips, sticky tape and string, and staffed by a cast of characters out of *Carry On* films. I had been literally crying with laughter one night a few months earlier as they took it in turns with their wonderful anecdotes; now I hoped David's tales might jog Kim's memory, and perhaps enough would come back to him to be able to tell a few of his own. David told us some of the latest farces but he was so shocked that the fizz had gone out of his stories. Nothing seemed so funny any more.

He took Kim for a walk around the block – the garden was becoming too small as an exercise yard – and came back jokingly to tell me the fellow was a liability. While out they had come across a man walking his dog and Kim had bent to stroke the Alsatian saying "nice pussy". The owner had thought Kim was some wise-cracking yob and was not amused.

Duncan came round later that evening after a twelve-hour shift in a television news room with another starting at nine the next morning, so he was not his usual merry self either. By supper time Kim was too exhausted by the rigours of the day to be able to do anything but eat, and even then not very much. It was a flat evening, with David in shock, Duncan shattered, Kim exhausted and me desperately trying to entertain

David and Duncan and look after Kim. Afterwards Duncan told me it was the first time he saw me beginning to go under, but he was helpless to do anything about it.

The person I was most concerned about was David. Kim had been like an elder brother to him and David had put him on something of a pedestal; suddenly to see him unable to look after himself and seemingly incapable of even thinking properly, then playing the fool as a way of putting people at their ease, was just too much for him. A few days later I received a note from him apologising for his behaviour. Quite unnecessary. Not only had he not done anything overt, it had been my insensitivity that had caused the situation: I had not warned him properly. From Kim's point of view the visit had not been in vain: fragments of memories from his Swansea Sound days had returned and he even started doing an impersonation of one of the characters he had known down there.

That Sunday morning Kim was featured in the *Sunday Times*. As I lay in the Greek hospital waiting for the air ambulance to be sent I had sworn vengeance on Medex, the holiday insurance company. As the drama of the moment had receded and I was left with the job of looking after Kim, the fire had rather gone out of me, but Kim's sister Susan had spurred me on. I also knew I would never forgive myself if I heard of a similar case in the future in which the delay caused by the deliberations of those men over whether to spend the money proved fatal – as it could have done with Kim. Some fuss in the papers and maybe the planes would fly that summer, and no one would have to go through what I went through. So I rang a friend of mine on the *Sunday Times*, Simon Freeman, and told him the story. And it was duly printed.

That Sunday Kim read the article over and over again; he was so proud to be in the paper, and have his picture on it, however shockingly gaunt he looked. He kept on reading it aloud, missing out the technical bits but glorying in the paragraphs which mentioned his name. He particularly liked being called a young television reporter, partly because he was still not convinced he had ever been one, partly because it sounded rather glamorous. Another reason he kept going back to it was that he could not remember he had already read it; each time he would show the same amazement at seeing himself in the papers and read out the same paragraphs with awe. My patience began to wear out, but his pleasure in continually rereading the article did not pall.

We went for lunch at Amanda's that day. She had promised faithfully she would not have another turn about doing the cooking, and although she had not quite kept the promise, at least what she managed to produce was edible.

Kim was introduced to Ken the kitten, or Ken the chicken as he insisted on calling him. Poor Kim would gently stroke Ken only to be rewarded by a vicious scratch. He would hold out his hand and say piteously: "The chicken's made me bleed."

When I drove him back to the hospital that evening I asked him what he remembered about the weekend. He held up his hand and showed me the scratches. For the first time he had been able to remember an incident which had happened more than an hour earlier, and typically it was one which had caused him pain. The next jump in progress – remembering an incident for a few days – concerned walking in the gardens in front of the hospital when a pigeon shat on his head. A tale he told for days but no longer remembers.

That day, also for the first time, he minded going back into hospital. As we walked into the ward he turned to me and asked what we were doing. I told him I was taking him back to his bed for the week.

"Don't make silly jokes. Let's go home."

"I'm serious, Kim, you have to stay here."

"Why? There's nothing wrong with me. I want to go home."

My stomach turned over. Kim was right. I had to ask myself the question. Why was Kim still in hospital? That week I started wading through the bureaucracy to find a way of getting him out.

Chapter 6
RED TAPE

It was now almost two months since the accident. Kim had long-term neurological problems but was on a ward for acute cases. His environment was becoming progressively more unsatisfactory. His needs had outgrown the hospital's facilities.

The only medication he was taking were Phenytoin tablets to prevent epilepsy attacks, a common side effect of head injuries. Kim had not had an attack, but while his blood gas levels were still unstable the doctors thought it wise to keep him on them, the better-safe-than-sorry principle. The medication was not tying him to the hospital.

Kim was beginning to show improvement only when he came home and would slump down again as soon as he was back in hospital. I mentally charted his progress weekend by weekend, and on each visit home he would manage to do something new, remember something for slightly longer or recall another event from his past, but during the weekdays he just seemed to stay the same.

It was not surprising. He needed constant stimulation and the hospital could not provide it. The nurses would spend as much time as possible by his bed talking to him, even taking him for walks in the square outside, but they could do that only if it was a quiet day on the ward.

He now had daily speech therapy, occupational therapy and physiotherapy but at the most only an hour of each. They were all good for him, but not enough. I was worried that time was being wasted. I knew that time was important in a brain injury, as the greatest progress was at the beginning. Sister Thorman had told me that Kim would reach a plateau in hospital, and then it would be for him to go somewhere else. I reckoned he had reached his plateau and the time had come.

The nurses and I were agreed that I could not have him at home all day and look after him by myself. It was a recipe for disaster because I was too involved and would not be able to show the impersonal patience that was needed. By the same token, he could not go to his parents in Bristol; that would anyway cut himself off from his life in London which I felt was desperately important to him as he began to recover. He needed proper intensive rehabilitation therapy, somewhere he could go or someone who would come to him. I even wondered if it would be possible to organise a rota of friends to do recommended exercises with him.

He was becoming quite a handful on the ward, always playing up to the nurses so they never knew whether he was joking or serious. One day his consultant Mr Hayward asked him where he got the name Sabido from.

"From my father, I hope," came the instant reply, leaving Mr Hayward dumbfounded and the nurses desperately trying to keep a straight face.

Another time his friend Andrew Burn was down visiting from Birmingham and they were in a nearby tea shop when Louise walked in. Kim called her over and asked if she was a nurse.

"Yes," she smilingly replied.

"Well, bugger off then." And he and Andrew both guffawed with laughter.

He was beginning to get lost more often as his wanderings took him further afield in the hospital, and he would have to be brought back from other wards, which was increasing the pressure on the nurses.

He still had a lot of visitors so at least he was getting stimulation from them. Most people had been in enough times to be able to slip easily onto Kim's wavelength and joke along with him. He still did not know who anyone was and was astonishingly rude, but he was quite fun to be with. It was debatable whether he was ever going to be able to get back to work, but it was difficult to feel sorry for him because he made such a determined effort to enjoy himself and keep everybody else amused.

The only positive aspect to the ward was the presence of John Gibbon. He was a maths lecturer who had come in for a back operation. He remembers on first being admitted a breathless nurse telling him that "there is an ITN reporter on the ward and lots of famous people visit him". It did not take him long to work out who it was as he saw the long stream of visitors going to Kim's bed at the end of the ward.

The morning after his operation he watched Kim walk through the doorway and suddenly Sister Kennedy shouted, "Oh no, nurse, he's gone walkabout again." She and the nurse rushed after him and reappeared five minutes later clutching Kim, who was wearing bright green socks and grinning inanely.

A few nights later Kim suddenly got out of his bed, sped over to Samer, stole one of his bananas and bolted it in two mouthfuls. Samer's mother started shouting at him in Arabic, presumably telling him to eat his own bloody bananas. Kim then could not find his own bed, so John shouted directions, "Right a bit, left a bit. No, no, that's Graham's bed, you fool." That was the beginning of their friendship.

John was so bored by his complete immobility, for he had to stay in bed for seven days after the operation, and so desperate to fill in the long hours between his wife's daily visits that he began to devise problems for Kim to solve and have long conversations with him, patiently keeping him to the point and putting up with the constant repetitions such an activity involved. It was good for Kim to have a proper friend on the ward, for however short a time – somebody he could chatter to outside visiting hours. It made me slightly less concerned about Kim's immediate welfare and more patient as I waited for the slow hospital wheels to turn. When John was able to move again they would take turns together round the gardens in the front – it was during one of these circuits that Kim was subjected to the pigeon droppings.

It was a time when I needed all my energy and patience to push for Kim's next move, but over the next four weeks other demands were going to be made on me.

My contract at Diverse finished in four weeks' time. I had been pregnant when I was originally given it, and it took me up until a few months before the baby was born. When I had had my miscarriage, my boss David Graham had written to me telling me to take time off, but saying he was looking forward to seeing me again. I had intended to renegotiate my contract after I returned from holiday, to finish in November like everybody else on contract. I had assumed it would just be a formality. However the accident meant I had never got it extended.

Barry Flynn, one of the union people at work, rang me to say they did not intend to extend it. I was horrified. To lose my job as well as everything else just seemed too much. Barry said I had the full support of all the union people there and advised me to come back to work – with my presence it would be more embarrassing not to renew my contract.

I did not want to go back to work. I was always exhausted when I was there. I was not sure how I was going to cope, but I asked Barry to tell them I was returning the following Monday.I then rang Duncan to ask him if I could do a few days at *City Limits*, to prepare myself for the world of work.

While I still had some time and energy left I made an appointment with the hospital social worker to discuss the options for Kim once he was out of the hospital. The social worker was extremely nice but the conversation was rather depressing. He had not seen Kim, so at first he suggested someone coming round to do the shopping for him twice a week when he was at home. I told him Kim would need constant supervision. So he suggested an old people's day centre. He was not trying to be horrible but I almost cried at the thought of Kim being sent every day to one of those stultifying places. At best they are somewhere for old people to go and entertain themselves; they are not for making somebody better. Not only would Kim have disliked it, the day centre would not have been able to deal with him because of his tendency to wander and his need to be kept constantly occupied. In comparison the ward appeared ideal: at least Kim was relatively happy with lots of nice nurses and many visitors to stop him from being too bored. I was shocked at the limited aftercare facilities and wondered how most brain-damaged people did get better.

The social worker said he would visit Kim for himself to see just what the problems were and then at the weekly conference held to assess every patient they could discuss his future. He warned me nothing would happen fast.

The conference decided Kim needed to be sent to the rehabilitation centre attached to the hospital, which was in Finchley in North London. Kim's name had been put on the waiting list. I thought this was a very good idea because it gave us a few weeks or possibly months for Kim to recover further before a final decision about his future had to be made, and before I had to have sole responsibility for him. It was now just a matter of waiting.

The three days I did at *City Limits* were among the happiest working days I have ever done. I had been slightly nervous about working for Duncan because some people change at work. But it was a lovely relaxed place and very friendly. I was given enough work to keep me busy but not so much that I felt bogged down.

Unfortunately it made going back to Diverse even more difficult; that office was anything but happy and relaxed. Even before the accident I had tried to work away from the office as much as possible because I had found the atmosphere so oppressive.

David Graham called me in on my first morning to tell me how sorry he was about everything that had happened, and asked me about Kim's progress. He said he had worried a lot about the two of us. I took his concern as a sign that there had just been a misunderstanding about my contract, because obviously I desperately needed a job. Everybody was terribly nice to me and treated me like the fragile flower I felt myself to be but the internecine warfare in the office continued around me as ever. I just did my work and left the office as soon as possible to go and see Kim.

One afternoon I walked in to see him and found chaos. Kim's sister Susan was there with Jon Snow from ITN, who had just returned from covering the Pope in Poland and had come to see Kim before he even went into ITN, and Ian Parkinson – the third of the terrible trio at Swansea Sound.

Ian told me he had only just found out about the accident: for the last couple of months people had come up to him at the BBC asking after Kim, and he had assumed they were just enquiring about his progress at ITN and had blithely told everybody that he was fine. This was his first opportunity to visit Kim since he had heard the bad news that morning. I told him that with his nose for news I would never employ him as a journalist. (To be fair, much later he managed to hear about the birth of our baby in a London hospital while he was in Dallas, Texas, and sent off immediate congratulations.)

What was so awful that afternoon was that Kim was just playing the fool. He apparently did not know who anybody was, not even me or Susan (he dubbed us both Veronica and guffawed whenever he said it). He kept on burbling nonsense and when Graham in the next bed gave one of his grumbling coughs Kim would shout: "Get an ambulance. There's a man dying here." He was a child showing off.

We spent ages trying to get him to remember Jon's name, with lots of clues about cold weather and skiing, but he was determined to keep up the façade of looniness. When Jon got ready to go he told Kim he would be in to see him at the weekend, and jokingly wagged a finger telling him he had better know his name by then. When I told Jon that Kim always came home at the weekends we were invited to Sunday supper.

As we drove to Jon's house that weekend I made Kim repeat who we were going to dinner with: Jon Snow, Jon Snow, Jon Snow. Even standing on the doorstep when I rang the bell I reminded him, and when Jon opened the door I turned to Kim with a flourish saying, "Who's this?"

On cue Kim replied, "Jon Snow."

Jon smiled appreciatively and said we had obviously been practising.

Inside was his girlfriend Madeleine. Becoming a friend of hers has been one of the benefits of the accident. In the months to come the four of us spent many evenings together, and I always came away feeling calmer and more relaxed. Not only did we have a good time with Jon entertaining us with anecdotes of his doings, but I always felt able to offload the troubles of the moment by discussing them, and as Kim's progress was left more and more up to me I would thrash out the options with the two of them. Madeleine asked penetrating questions, revealing her training as a barrister, and by the end of an evening just by answering her I would have worked out a lot of the problems for myself. Madeleine agreed that I had a terrible responsibility because only results could reveal whether I had taken the wrong or right decision, and by then it would be too late to change course.

She was also wonderful with Kim. With a quiet self-effacing manner which inspired confidence she talked to him and took an interest in what he was saying. She had quite enough problems of her own to contend with: her hair was coming out in lumps and the doctors had no idea whether she would go bald. It was obviously stress-related because it started after she went back to work at the end of her maternity leave a few months earlier. She had a hard job working at the Children's Legal Centre which she had helped to set up a few years earlier, was the mother of a young child, Leila, and went out with Jon who was quite hard work himself.

That first evening was particularly good. Jon made it clear we had been invited out for a proper dinner. The table was laid with silver cutlery, linen tablecloth and glasses for wine, mineral water and brandy. A three-course meal was served. Kim responded to the propriety of it all by being better behaved than ever. It was the first proper dinner we had been invited out to and at times during that evening I felt we were like any other couple, just out to dinner with friends, not pathetic souls limping from day to day. Jon had decided it was going to be a fun, ordinary evening and his will was strong enough to pull us all into the fantasy.

When I took Kim back to hospital that Monday morning, one of the nurses took me aside and asked how I thought he was progressing. I said he seemed to be getting on fine. She told me that in the hospital he appeared to have come to halt. He was still getting lost all the time and had difficulty finding the loo. I was quite worried by her words because by this time he had sorted out the geography of our house. I spoke to Sister Thorman about getting him out and she just said I had to be patient, his turn to go to Finchley would come.

That day Amanda visited him and rang me at home in the evening to tell me how different he was from the person she had seen at the weekend. All his sparkiness had gone.

Kim was a constant nagging worry while I was at work. He was becoming much more demanding. He had realised there was a telephone on the ward and had started ringing people, with the help of John Gibbon. He most often called his parents because theirs was the only number he knew, and he would worry them terribly as he would plead with them to get him out. He also kept wanting to get hold of ITN, so I asked John to get him to ring me instead, but his calls just made me feel increasingly impotent.

To me Kim seemed desperate and unhappy, but John said that for the most part on the ward he seemed fine and John still remembers many of the funny incidents. Kim had played John the ITN tape he had been given by Joan Thirkettle, which John found quite fascinating. Ten minutes later Kim was back to tell him about a tape he had just found. John heard it four times that day and over twenty times by the end of the week. He knew it off by heart.

John found his attitude to visitors quite novel. Most were greeted by Kim with, "Who are you? Never heard of you." Occasionally Kim would nod and smile politely and chat, then after the visitor had gone John would ask who it was and Kim would just shrug and say, "Haven't a clue."

One afternoon when Jon Snow called round the three of them went for a walk in the square. Jon asked John how Kim was getting on, then turned to Kim and said, "What's my name?" The response was "Frank – or is it Brian?" John said the look on Jon's face was a picture of conflicting emotions: hurt pride, understanding laughter and confusion.

One lunchtime Kim had a succession of four visitors and when John asked how he had enjoyed talking to so many people Kim said, "Which people?"

John told him there had been four people there, including two good-looking women.

"Really?" said Kim. "They never talked to me. Who did they come to see?"

"You, you fool. You've spent two hours talking to friends and you can't remember a thing. Tell me, where did those two punnets of strawberries come from?"

"What strawberries?" said Kim.

"The ones you're eating."

"Scarlett brought them yesterday."

"No she didn't. They came at lunchtime from a friend."

"Which friend? Nobody came to see me."

This conversation went on for about half an hour, during which time Kim managed to eat most of the strawberries.

As a result of this scrambling of visits and incidents, combined with the telescoping of time and events, Kim would wake in the night and remember visitors who had been there at lunchtime. He would then insist to the night nurses that two men from ITN were in the waiting-room. It took a long talk and a cup of tea to convince him that perhaps the men really had been there but had had to leave on urgent business.

John often found Kim's strange behaviour hilarious. At this time his physiotherapist was called Barbara, but he could never remember her name. So John tried to train him to say, "Hello, Barbara, how are you?", to please her. For half an hour they practised until Kim had it off pat. They then went to the lift to go to the gym. The doors opened and there stood Matron in all her glory. Kim fixed her with a beady eye and said, "Hello, Barbara. How are you?"

Her face froze for a moment then broke into a big grin when she realised who he was. He completely forgot his lines when they got to the real Barbara.

In the gym John was learning how to walk again but Kim had outgrown most of the exercises so they used to put him on the exercise bicycle and make him pedal away to tone his muscles and use up some of his excess energy. One day John was on the mat doing his exercises when a familiar voice shouted above the noise: "You're all condemned."

He looked up to see Kim in his bright green socks pedalling away madly, shouting rude comments at the top of his voice. He announced that the staff were prison warders and told his fellow patients who were contorting themselves in their exercises that they could be arrested for their postures. John was laughing so much the tears were streaming down his face. The staff took this as proof that Kim no longer needed physiotherapy. So it was his last visit to the gym, or the factory as he always called it.

His code words made sense if one tried to look through his eyes, or his brain. John could understand why he called the gym a factory because he said it looked like a scene from a Breughel painting with people limping, rolling, hobbling and riding all over the place. When John asked him about his job at ITN, Kim said he went visiting energy platforms, which John translated as hot spots, in the news sense, which again made sense.

Once when he was recording his day for his occupational therapist he wrote: "Scarlet Macwine visited me." To this day John thinks of me as Scarlett Macwine. It was to take months before Kim relearnt to spell my name.

Sometimes John felt Kim was more aware than he pretended to be. One morning he finished his breakfast and went to the loo. His tray was removed and when he returned he complained that he had not had any breakfast. Everybody assured him he had already eaten it. However he insisted he had not and the nurses finally gave in and served him a second one. John is still certain Kim was just having them on, to get more food.

During the last few days John was on the ward, he and Kim would often go to a nearby tea shop. Kim would drink endless cups of tea and eat lots of pastries while John asked him questions about his travels for IRN and ITN. One afternoon Kim told him all about a long trip to Africa, what he did there and the countries he visited. John was very impressed until I told him Kim had never been to the continent.

On the way back he addressed a tree as "Brian", mistaking it for one of his ITN colleagues because of his bad eyesight.

His sense of surroundings was quite frighteningly absent. One day he got into bed in one of the women's wards downstairs, thinking it was his own. Wrong floor, wrong ward, wrong bed.

Every time John wandered over to Kim's bed to speak to him, Kim would warmly greet him as if he were a new visitor – even though it could have been the fortieth time that day they had talked.

When John was discharged I knew I had to act. My last excuse for inactivity had gone. It was now imperative that Kim be taken away from the ward, otherwise I could envisage him still there at Christmas, vegetating. A child minder I knew was prepared to look after him for a while. She was very patient and I had noticed that Kim was at his best with children. She was also a trained nurse.

I rang Mr Hayward, explained I was desperate to get Kim out of the hospital and told him of the arrangements I had made. He was very understanding and amenable and we agreed that Kim would leave in two weeks.

Then suddenly there was a place at the rehabilitation centre at Finchley. Jo, Kim's occupational therapist, was so worried about Kim not receiving structured therapy when he left that she had persuaded Finchley to take him on. He did not jump any queue, there was no shortage of places at Finchley, the staff there just had not wanted him because they thought he would be too troublesome.

I was amazed to learn from John Gibbon that the nurses at the National regarded me as a bit of an ogre because of my fight to get Kim out. I had always felt guilty about not pushing hard enough for him and just letting time pass for so long.

Most people obviously leave it up to the "professionals" to decide what is best, but the creaking administration of the NHS is so slow-moving it needs to be kicked into action to make sure patients receive the best it can provide. To me Kim was the most important person in the world and his recovery was top priority, but to the hospital Kim was one of the many people who would have done better somewhere else but as long as he was pleasant on the ward, moving him was not a priority. Medically he was fine and some rehabilitation was being done, so he was not actually getting worse. I am a reasonably articulate middle-class woman, and was used to questioning authority and getting what I wanted, and still it took up a great deal of time and energy. I felt sorry for people without my advantages. I now know I should have gone straight to Mr Hayward and something would have been done. Not because nobody else was trying, but because the wishes of a consultant are not ignored, while the wishes of a ward sister can be.

The immediate problem with Kim was finally solved, but it now looked as though I was going to lose my job. In spite of David Graham's words of sympathy to me he had decided not to renew my contract.

Part of the shocking hypocrisy about it all was that Diverse was supposed to be a radical television company in a new mould. But as far as its own industrial relations practices were concerned, it was a throwback. My case was just one of the many that year showing employees that the company could shed them at will. Their *Friday Alternative* programme was often extremely critical of ITN for its anti-union stories, so it was an irony that while ITN gave Kim constant emotional and financial security Diverse just pulled the rug from under my feet.

I went to see the industrial relations man who started muttering that the company was not in the business of providing jobs for life; but all I wanted was for my contract to run until November, which it would have done if I had not become pregnant. He told me that was hardly his fault if I had a miscarriage. He did stress that the action was not personal, but he could not allow my case to become a precedent so the union thought it could get any contract renewed. When he told me how bad he felt doing it, I grimly told him I had no sympathy to waste on him.

My contract ran out the day Kim was due to be discharged. The last weekend that he was in hospital and I was in work I took him to Bristol to see his parents. We travelled down by train because I thought a car journey would be too tiring for me, and Kim would definitely get bored and restless. It would be easier to keep him entertained on the train by chatting, doing puzzles or, if need be, just walking to and from the buffet car.

As well as wanting to see Kim, his mother hoped visiting Bristol would boost his progress and possibly provide a breakthrough to a full recovery. She thought one of the reasons his memory of the past was showing so little improvement compared to his immediate, short-term memory was because there was nothing concrete for it to hook onto. When he came home at the weekends it was to a relatively strange house which held no memories because it had been bought so soon before the accident. His brothers and Susan had also all moved within the last year, so their houses were clean of familiarity; but his parents' house was the one he had been brought up in. Perhaps by seeing the people he had known all his life in their correct setting something would be jogged.

His mother was right but not as dramatically as she had hoped. For the first time he obviously knew a place and was sure of the geography of both house and garden. It was a hot summer's weekend and we spent Saturday and Sunday out in the garden with Kim's mother keeping up a virtual conveyer belt of food to us. Kim was happy to be at home and his childhood came flooding back. The last ten years were still mostly blank, so much so that he could not believe he was twenty-eight and still thought of himself as eighteen. That evening his mother brought out the family snapshot album and the two of them told me about every photo.

Kim's brother Roger had picked us up from the station, and he and his wife Susan and their two children, Hannah and baby William, also spent the weekend with us. Hannah had always been particularly fond of Kim and now for two blissful days she had him at her beck and call. For hours they played hide and seek and catch; we could hear their squeals as they chased each other round the garden. William was five months old; as I held him I could only think of the baby I had lost and how things might have been. Sue was wonderful. She knew all too tragically about loss: she had had a baby between Hannah and William who had died.

In many respects Kim behaved normally that weekend. For much of the time we could kid ourselves the improvement had been such that there were only a few minor problems left, as long as we forgot about the Kim we had known before the accident. Then suddenly he would say something which would demonstrate his frightening loss of memory. He had five baths over those two days, because he kept on forgetting he had just had one, but remembering he had been intending to have one he would go upstairs and run himself another. His mother became quite upset as he flatly denied having just had one. By mid-morning on Sunday he thought we had only been there a few hours; he remembered nothing of the day before.

The previous night we had been put in a spare room rather than Kim's old bedroom because there were two beds in it. He woke, as always, for his middle-of-the-night pee and went to the bathroom alone because he knew where it was. When he did not return I went looking for him and found him in his old bedroom trying to get into an unmade bed. After a brief argument I persuaded him that he had the wrong room and took him back to bed. He looked horrified when I started getting back into my own bed and told me I was not allowed to sleep there. I climbed into bed regardless and he hissed at me that his mother would be furious if she found out. I told him she knew and had put us in the room together. He would not believe me and would not be content until I promised to take all the responsibility and blame.

His conviction that he was an adolescent was causing a few problems for our relationship. At times he said I was his sister as a way of giving me an important place in his life, though by doing this he only confused himself because he knew he had only one sister, Susan. He sometimes tried to overcome this problem by calling me Susan, but that was equally unsatisfactory.

During the day he seemed quite happy for us to go about together, but at night he found it odd to sleep in the same bed as me. We often had arguments about it. I would have been happy to sleep separately but because of his wanderings Kim could not be left to spend the night alone; as long as we were in the same bed I was a light enough sleeper always to wake when Kim got out of bed.

The crunch came just after he left hospital. We had been down to Winchester for the day to see his sister Susan and her family and returned quite late. Walking home from the tube station he told me he owned a house round here. I agreed and said that was where we were going, to the house where we lived together. He sternly told me we did not live together, he lived in a house without me. We went on arguing until we reached home, and he told me this was not the house he was thinking of, he lived in another one.

I explained our situation: I was his girlfriend and we lived together. Not wanting to hurt me he kindly told me that he liked me very much but he did not want to have a serious relationship with a girl just yet, and he did not want to live with me. I told him he did not have much choice in the matter for the moment because he needed looking after; but I assured him if he still felt like that when he was better he need no longer live with me. We agreed on that compromise.

At the end of the Bristol weekend Roger drove us to the station and in true British Rail summer weekend fashion the train was running about an hour late. To kill time Roger drove us to some nearby playing fields to watch cricket and on the way we stopped at a garage where I bought Kim a watch.

I hoped his would make him aware of time passing and give the day a structure. It could even aid his memory to know at what time things happened. It was also a way to get round the nurses always asking him the date when they did their checks on him. Not surprisingly he never knew, nor did he know the day of the week in that limbo world of hospital where most long-stay patients find the days and weeks drift into each other. I taught him how to tell the date and the time by pushing a button on his watch, so he would be able to answer the questions correctly. Even this small short cut took a long time to master. At first I always had to remind him to look at his watch; then he needed help to work out that the seventh month was July, counting up the months on his fingers. By the time he had them in the correct order he would forget he had to stop at the seventh. So we began again. When he finally had all that sorted out he would often go wrong on the year. But it helped. Weeks later, when he had finally mastered it, it gave him a sense of achievement.

His own watch had come off in the crash. While he was still on the ventilator I was sitting in his room with Susan fishing for something in my handbag when I came across it – I had been given it to hold as we lay on the road after the accident. I showed it to Susan, pointing out where the watchband had been severed by the impact, and commented on the fact that, incredibly, it was still keeping perfect time even though it was only a cheap £2.99 garage watch. When Kim came off the ventilator, his speech therapist, Fiona, spent some time with him every day trying to encourage him to talk. She did this with picture cards, getting him to find the right word to identify the object, which was a tremendous effort, and then talk about it, which took a lot of encouragement from Fiona. When he was shown a picture of a watch he spontaneously told her his own had been broken in the accident. Fiona was amazed, particularly when I corroborated the story. We agreed it was unlikely he remembered the actual incident, but must have been recalling my conversation with Susan weeks earlier. By the next day he did not know he had ever had a watch.

On the Monday after we returned from Bristol Kim's mother rang him at the hospital for a chat. He remembered nothing about the weekend and would not believe he had been to Bristol.

My last week at Diverse was one of the worst I have ever had. A great deal of it was spent in union meetings and negotiations.

It was such an awful place to work that a part of me was glad to be getting out. The problem was my next move. It would be difficult to get another job. I would sink under depression if my life just revolved around looking after Kim, but I did not feel dynamic enough to go out and persuade an employer I would be a good prospect. The outlook was depressing.

Parliament was due to debate hanging and the programme had decided to get someone who supported the death penalty to meet a convicted murderer. I had to meet a man who had been in a condemned cell for twenty-seven days before his sentence was commuted on appeal in the days before hanging was abolished and take him to meet a woman who wanted the death penalty brought back.

The alleged murderer and I took a train to Ipswich and back for the meeting and for those hours I almost forgot all the awful things that were happening to me. He was one of the most pleasant people I had ever met. He convinced me that he had not taken part in the armed robbery he was convicted of, let alone fired the gun, but he had spent seventeen years in prison. He showed me the press cuttings that had been written about him while he was waiting to die in the condemned cell, before he won his appeal. Real gutter press stuff about the nastiest man in Britain, and how he would die a lonely abandoned man because his wife had left him during the trial. He felt that one of the reasons his sentence had been cut on appeal rather than the case overturned was the strength of feeling generated by the newspaper articles. I have never seen him again but during those hours together we told each other all about our lives, and he was very sympathetic about my plight.

I had to go back and edit the piece that night so I quickly visited Kim on the way back. The nurses were being particularly wonderful to me because they felt so sorry for me losing my job. Kim obviously sensed something was up because he kept on trying to stop me leaving.

I arrived at Diverse and started talking to Anna Coote. Within half an hour I was in hysterical tears. For the first time since the accident I thought I had reached breaking point. She took over the editing and I went home to cry myself out.

I went back to Diverse to pick up my things the next day. When David Graham came up to me and asked after Kim, I just turned on my heel and walked out.

I went to the hospital to pick up Kim, taking in a few boxes of chocolates as a thank you to the nurses. We cracked open a bottle of champagne which Max Hastings, who was in the Falklands with Kim, had had delivered to the hospital. I was not going to let myself think of the future, I just made myself be happy because Kim was coming home. I was almost sad to go, the nurses had been so kind. Many of them told me the ward was just not going to be the same without him.

Chapter 7
FINCHLEY

Kim started at Finchley Rehabilitation Centre the Wednesday after he left hospital, two and a half months after the accident. I had been asked to accompany him and stay with him for the three days of that first week, so I could help him find his way around and get him used to the routine.

The Centre was an imposing Victorian house set in well-kept gardens which, although only yards from the thunder of articulated lorries pounding up the Finchley High Road, were an enclave of quiet as the noise of traffic was deadened by the surround of high bushes. Most of the other patients were suffering from multiple sclerosis or spinal problems rather than head injuries, and their disabilities dictated the slow pace which gave an aura of peace to the place.

The facilities inside the house were basic, with dormitories for the patients, all of whom, with the exception of Kim, were residential. He was, however, given a bed which he could use when he felt tired during the day. The occupational therapy department, where Kim would spend most of his time, was a prefabricated annexe to the main building so that everything was conveniently placed on the ground floor. During those summer weeks it was light and airy.

The day room, where Kim spent his time between therapy sessions, was in the main part of the house. It was a dark room in spite of the windows and door leading out into the garden, with heavy, hard-wearing old furniture and a small bookcase of old-fashioned books, few of which I had heard of and most of which I was sure had been out of print for years. There was also a radio which for those weeks appeared permanently tuned to Radio Two. Down the corridor was the dining-room, serving up the usual over-cooked institution food.

I had hoped for some recreational facilities but NHS resources only stretched to the most basic: there was provision for the exercise of those physically handicapped but nothing for able-bodied Kim.

Stella Doble was Kim's occupational therapist – I remembered her from Queen's Square where she had given Kim his first few sessions before she transferred to Finchley. Neither of us was sure whether Kim recognised her, although he said he did remember her. She told me Kim would have two occupational therapy sessions a day, an hour in the morning and an hour in the afternoon; the rest of the time he would be expected to keep himself occupied and amused. I did not think this was enough, but realised he could not expect to receive attention all day and at least for those two hours he had Stella's undivided attention, for they were individual sessions. At this stage he could not just be left to get on with things – he would forget what he was supposed to be getting on with. The sessions gradually became all-morning and all-afternoon ones and he learned to work on his own: answering general knowledge questions from quiz books, filling in the events of the night before in his diary, or recalling the pertinent parts of articles in the *Daily Mirror*, which he brought in every day to make his memory exercises relevant to his needs and keep up some basic knowledge of current affairs.

Stella freely admitted she had never dealt with problems like Kim's before; when Kim first received therapy in Queen's Square he was in such a state it was more a matter of assessing the degree of impairment than trying therapeutically to deal with it. She intended to use what she thought were appropriate exercises, but told me she would welcome any suggestions, particularly concerning skills he would need at work. For all her modesty she achieved great progress with Kim; by the time he left in early September he had a limited independence, was able to communicate more easily and had developed a few tricks to aid his memory.

That first day I was just worried there was not enough for Kim to do. However I was impressed with what occupational therapy there was. The morning session was spent assessing Kim: he had to pick the odd one out from groups of objects, assemble different coloured blocks in a pattern, do some writing and even some easy mental arithmetic. Stella and I both remembered when she had first done this assessment back in Queen's Square: he could manage nothing and finally motioned he had given up by laying his head on the desk and closing his eyes. This time he found difficulty only with problems which involved his memory.

Stella decided Kim should make his own elevenses and proceeded to demonstrate how to make a pot of tea. She showed him where the cups and tea bags were, how to switch on the electric kettle, and then gave him the teapot. When the kettle boiled he poured a little water into the pot; she stopped him and told him he had forgotten the tea. He looked up perplexed and told her he was warming the pot. We learned there were some things Kim did not need teaching.

In the afternoon he played a simple memory game. A tray with four items on it was shown to him, then one of them was removed and he had to say what it was. A good exercise, but hard work for both Kim and Stella. Kim's first problem was that he did not know the names of the objects. A pencil, a comb, a pen top and a paper clip would be put on the tray, then the first five minutes would be spent trying to identify them. He knew what they all were, but could not find the correct word. Thinking hard and trying desperately to remember just resulted in a lot of wild guesses so Stella tried a new tack. She made Kim describe the object and what was done with it, and in the flow of speech the word would come back, often unnoticed. He would, for example, talk about combing his hair, and Stella would have to stop him and say: so this is a. . . .? Then Kim would get it right. From then on I used this method often with Kim. By the time he had managed to find the word for the last item on the tray, he would have forgotten what the first one was called, so the exercise would have to be repeated, until finally he could say all four easily. When the tray was removed and an item taken away, he would once again forget all the names of the things on the tray, and have no idea what had been taken away. He played the game three or four times that afternoon and not once did Stella display the slightest sign of impatience. It showed how good it was that he was not at home all day: I would have been screaming at him. But at the end of the day I did wonder if the Centre really was the right place for him. He would spend most of his time there just sitting around and the air of languor hanging over everybody was stultifying.

In this slightly despondent mood I received a call from Janis, the secretary of the East London group of Headway, the association for people with head injuries, who had been put on to me by a friend of Duncan's. I desperately felt the need to talk to someone who understood what I was going through and Headway provided this sort of service. I spilled out all my worries and told her just how difficult I was finding living constantly with this burden. It was the first time I felt I could honestly talk about how tough I was finding everything. I did not want to be disloyal, but as Janis was almost a professional counsellor it was not like telling tales. I had been slightly worried about myself and how much longer I would be able to cope, but having Janis to pour it out to immediately made the problem more manageable.

She was a speech therapist at a rehabilitation unit in Hackney specialising in head injuries, and asked why Kim was not in there. She told me a lot about the unit which seemed almost custom-made for him, for they concentrated on young people. I wondered why nobody at Queen's Square had mentioned it to me. We even lived in the borough of Hackney, so the red tape would have been minimal. She said they took people within days of coming off the ventilator, as soon as they were physically stable enough to leave hospital, believing the earlier intensive rehabilitation was started the greater the chances of recovery. I was so angry with myself for not having done my homework properly and allowing the hospital to put forward the options rather than discovering them myself, and for not having contacted Headway myself but just letting Duncan organise it, so precious weeks had passed. I worried about how much Kim had lost by not being at the Hackney unit from the beginning. Rather than crying over spilt milk, Janis suggested I got him there as soon as possible.

There was one problem: it was residential, and I thought that now Kim had had a taste of living at home he would not want to stay in another institution. I told her I would have to discuss it with him. Earlier in the conversation I had said that living with Kim was like being with a child; Janis hearkened back to this and said that, like a child, Kim did not know what was best for him, so I should not take his view too seriously. I disagreed. Kim might have the dependency of a child but he did not think like one and it was extremely important I did not treat him as one. I understood why Kim liked living at home: he was more in control and not bound by the parameters of an imposed regime. No one wants to spend time in an institution. She agreed to see if an exception could be made in his case, but meanwhile suggested Kim and I should look round the place and perhaps he would change his mind.

Before we went to look round Stella told me that Fiona, Kim's speech therapist, had also been worried about Kim's rehabilitation, so had telephoned Barbara Wilson, the psychologist at the Rivermead Rehabilitation Unit in Oxford. I had been told about Rivermead while at Queen's Square, the best memory place in Britain, but when attempts were made to get Kim admitted we were told there was a six-month waiting list for patients from outside the Oxfordshire Health Authority. He was put on the waiting list, but I hoped that in six months' time he would no longer need it. (The discreet silence which greeted this remark showed my prognosis was on the optimistic side.)

Barbara Wilson was a memory specialist and Kim's case interested her. As he was able-bodied she wondered if there was a way of making him a daily patient, then he could be admitted as soon as she had assessed him. Kim's brother Richard worked in Oxford and I was sure he would be willing to have him to stay with his family in Amersham, and could drop Kim off on his way to work. The hitch was that Barbara would be away in August, but she was quite willing to see him in early September.

This information took the urgency out of moving Kim from Finchley; chopping and changing him all over the place was not going to do any good at all. Janis had rung me to say Kim would have to live in the Hackney unit during the week, otherwise the other patients might feel he was receiving special treatment, though he could come home at the weekends. Kim had made it plain he wanted to live at home.

I had already made up my mind by the time we went to the Eastern Hospital, where Janis's unit was, and the visit confirmed it. The residential part was an enormous room with beds lining either side in military fashion and many of the inmates had severe physical as well as mental problems; nothing was going to persuade Kim this was preferable to living at home. I felt the stimulation he was getting outside his rehabilitation – friends coming round in the evenings, having to get himself up in the morning, choose what to wear, get dressed, all the everyday things we take for granted and he desperately needed to get used to was making up for anything which might be lacking at Finchley.

Janis put a fair amount of pressure on me, talking of the benefits Kim would get from intensive rehabilitation. I felt pulled and tugged every way and finally rang Barbara Wilson both to ask her advice and arrange a day when she could see Kim. Poor Barbara, having to deal with this neurotic woman almost out of her mind with worry. She agreed with me about the benefits of Kim being at home, and did not actually offer advice, but let me convince myself my instincts were right. I finally felt calm about my decision and I looked forward to her taking Kim on because I thought she would deal with all sides of him.

Janis accepted my final decision and still continued to be an ear into which I could pour out my troubles. She rang me often to keep a regular check on me, and we talked and talked. For the most part she was reassuring but always honest, and there were two matters she could not be completely reassuring about: whether Kim would ever fully recover and if our relationship would survive the strain. She was the only person to whom I confided my doubts on these questions, for I felt that talking about either was disloyal to Kim and could be counterproductive.

At this time Joan Thirkettle, who had made the ITN tape for Kim, did two very important things. First she arranged for ITN to pay for a taxi to take Kim to Finchley every day and bring him home and, second, she made an appointment for us to see a healer.

The taxi idea was marvellous. I did not take it up for a few weeks but when I did it freed me to work, as I could do none being tied to ferrying Kim around.

One morning there was a slight hitch when Kim was driven to a hospital he did not recognise. He told the driver he did not think this was the right place, but the driver, knowing of his condition, said he was certain he would recognise it once he was inside. Kim was so used to being wrong he did not question it, but once inside after the taxi had driven off, he knew he did not know where he was. Asking at reception he discovered he had been taken to the General Hospital at Finchley. After a lot of effort he managed to explain where he wanted to be. He was directed to a bus and found his way to the rehabilitation unit. I was extremely proud of him and relieved that however bad his memory, and at times his power of communication, at least his basic faculties were there and ultimately he could cope.

Another time his driver was stopped by a policeman for some alleged minor offence. Kim was furious and offered to be a defence witness if the case ever came to court. He became quite excited and told everybody about it, until the irony of the situation hit me and, giggling, I told him his credibility as a witness would be rather called into question when he was asked why he was in the taxi, and he would have to reply that his memory was so bad he could never remember where he was going.

More important than the taxis was the healer. Joan had taken me out to lunch while Kim was still in hospital and when the conversation turned to homeopathic medicine, I said I thought there was probably a lot in it. Later she came round to see me and asked if I would take Kim to a healer. I thought homeopathy was a rational alternative medical treatment but healing seemed to demand a leap of faith I was not sure I had. However, I felt no avenue should go unexplored and definitely did not want to appear to reject a kindness. Joan fixed up an appointment and I kept it. I was certain nothing would happen and thought we might even be turned away because I had no faith, but at least it would do no harm, and keep Joan happy.

It was a midday appointment so I asked if I could take Kim out to lunch from Finchley; I knew if I told the staff where we were really going they would think me a complete crank. The healer lived north of London and as we drove there Kim asked who we were going to see. I just said somebody wanted to talk to him (there was no point in raising false hopes) and he would have to answer her questions and do whatever she said. He groaned and said he was sick of answering questions. We got lost on the way there, and I almost took that as an omen and turned back, but eventually we arrived.

Beryl answered the door and was so very normal and warm-natured, with no hint of the occult, that I thought it would be pleasant just to spend some time with her, even if she could do nothing. She was probably in her late forties, a petite blonde with a ready smile. I presumed her husband had a good job, for she charged nothing for these consultations, saying it was a privilege to be able to help, yet lived in a beautiful large modern bungalow set in acres of parkland. The sitting-room, where she saw us, was expensively furnished with lots of velvet-covered chairs in pale shades of mauve, the walls and carpets in matching blues and pinks – all à la Barbara Cartland, I immediately thought, and later discovered the author was one of her patients.

She asked a few basic questions about the accident and Kim's current problems, then sat him on a stool in front of her, put her hands on his head and gently pressed his skull. For a few minutes she moved her hands around his cranium, gently pressing all the while. She said his brain was still healing and she could feel there was a lot wrong with it. Then she put her fingers over his eyes, for Kim had told her about his problems with double vision, and gently massaged his closed eyelids. Taking her hands away she told him to open his eyes.

"I can see," Kim gasped.

It was incredible. The lazy eye had disappeared. They were both normal again. It was only then I realised just how bad his eyes had been, by his happiness now at seeing the world as everybody else saw it. If she did nothing else, Beryl had achieved a breakthrough in just doing that. How could he remember things if he could not see them? Now he would be able to read, he would no longer suffer from terrible headaches, his progress was bound to take a leap. As I tried to express my gratitude she just modestly told me that eyes were easy, the optical nerve was near the surface so it responded well.

In spite of the near miracle I had just seen her perform, she was still worried about her ability to do very much for Kim. She said she was quite willing to try but she did not want to raise any false hopes as she had never dealt with this sort of problem before.

The healing of his eye was the first thing Kim was able to remember after the accident and marked the first step in the return of his memory functions.

When he saw Beryl again a week or so later he asked if this time she could fix his memory. She smiled sympathetically and gently told him that the brain healed very slowly, and although she could slightly accelerate the process, nothing dramatic was going to happen; he would have to be patient. Kim always felt better for seeing her, although he would often be so exhausted by the ten-minute session that he would spend much of the rest of the day asleep.

A few weeks later he complained of spasms in his arms emanating from his heart; they bothered him a lot but hospital tests could find nothing wrong. I was experiencing a similar sort of sensation with tingling up and down my arms and occasional numbness. Being a silent hypochondriac I decided it was multiple sclerosis and worried greatly but said nothing. At a Headway social, a physiotherapist told me we probably each had a trapped nerve, the result of the impact from falling off the bike, and unfortunately nothing could be done. On the next visit to Beryl, Kim told her about the problem, and I verified it, adding that I had it in a milder form. She too diagnosed it as a trapped nerve and massaged the area, then suggested exercises he could do to help it. She motioned to me to come and sit on the stool. I felt a bit of a fraud because this was Kim's session and I did not want to muscle in on it but I did want help with the nerve and also wondered what it felt like to be treated by her, because Kim could not describe the sensation. It was wonderful, like a champagne infusion. I could feel my muscles relax as she touched them, then she ran her finger up my spine causing a tingle right through me. There was magic in her fingers. The problem in my arms gradually got better over the next few days. Kim had to go a second time before he was cured because his was more serious.

Much later a friend of mine went to her with pelvic inflammatory disease which was so serious she had been on antibiotics most of the preceding year and had still spent a great deal of it in pain. She loved swimming, but as it exacerbated her condition she wondered if she would ever be able to do it again. After three sessions with Beryl she went on holiday feeling wonderful and she was able to swim a hundred lengths a day.

Beryl told me she had discovered her gift quite by accident. She used to calm her husband when he returned from a hard day at the office by massaging his skull and giving him a gin and tonic, always believing it was probably the drink which washed away his cares. One day a friend who was staying with them had a migraine attack, and Beryl's husband told her to give the woman a massage to make her better. Beryl was terribly embarrassed, but did as she was asked and to her surprise the pain went away. Then her daughter brought home a friend whose knee cartilage was causing him terrible pain. This time Beryl was a little cross about his hopes being raised, but once again her power worked. She realised she had the gift of healing. She started reading books about anatomy and physiology, and learned a lot from a chiropractor friend of hers, so that she could more knowledgeably apply her gift. She said she was sure many people unknowingly had it, but never had the time to notice. She stressed she could not work miracles or halt the ageing process, but she could relieve pain and heal.

My experience with Beryl completely convinced me of the power of healing. I am sure she did a great deal to help his brain to heal as well as the obvious improvement in his eyes and trapped nerve.

A remarkable woman.

Kim took a long time to like Finchley and for weeks he hated me leaving him there. When I woke him up in the mornings he would pretend to forget why he had to get up, then he would slowly have a shower, dress himself and have breakfast, while I continually chivvied him to hurry up. All the time he would be asking if he really had to go, until I finally got him into the car and drove him there. When we arrived he would burst into tears, which would trigger me off and we would both sit there sobbing until I pulled myself together, wiped our faces and sent him off.

I was so ready to burst into tears because I was finding life tough, having to cope with Kim and trying to find work. I kept my worries away from Kim as much as possible, but when a place which I thought would give me some casual work turned me down I just broke into uncontrollable sobs, saying to poor Kim that I would never get another job, nobody would hire me again and I was useless. He put his arms round me and told me he knew how wonderful I was and other people should appreciate what I had done for him. They were moving words but at the time I felt my commitment to Kim would put off any employer (as in fact it did); it might make me a better person but that is of little account in journalism. But his words did give me faith that when he needed to he was be able to give strength rather than rely on mine.

I told Stella about his crying, partly because she needed as much information about Kim as possible and partly because I hoped she might be able to offer some solutions. She said I should take it as a positive sign that he was becoming more aware of both his condition and his surroundings. During the day he showed no signs of unhappiness, in fact she had found his constant cheeriness rather unnerving. She did not want him to sink into a depression but was worried his tranquillity meant he did not realise there was anything wrong with him. This unhappiness was a sign that he was beginning to realise something was wrong, which meant he would work to overcome his problems. Later, when I told Barbara Wilson about it, she said bouts of tearfulness were common among people suffering from head injuries and, although difficult to deal with, were just part of the healing process.

One evening we returned, both rather overtired, from a second weekend in Bristol with his parents and he started talking in funny voices and cracking adolescent jokes. When I asked him to stop he told me he was trying to make me laugh. I told him I did not think the jokes were funny, but he just went on. He continued until I snapped and sharply told him to shut up. He promptly burst into tears and said he was just trying to make me laugh by telling jokes. If I laughed it meant I was happy. He wanted to make me happy. I felt so cruel and horrible I too burst into tears. Suddenly I had a vision of what it must be like for him: underneath the genial slow exterior was the old Kim, a successful television reporter, used to running his own life and shaping it for himself, now having to put up with being treated like a child, always being told what to do, performing fatuous exercises for Stella and putting up with it all with good humour because he did not know how else to cope. He desperately wanted people to like him and all he felt able to do was make people laugh, not caring if it was with him or at him; he had no idea of the admiration people had for the way he dealt with this terrifying situation. That night he had to comfort me, and he was even apologetic although it was me who had been insensitive; but I suppose he was used to crass insensitivity from me and everybody else.

As Kim began to settle into Finchley I started seriously looking for work. I rang up Colin Parkes, who was a duty editor at IRN and had written telling me to do just that if I needed to. He offered me two weeks of evening work, not particularly convenient hours but I knew he had made an effort to get them for me and I could arrange for other people to look after Kim.

Every evening when I left for work he would be in tears; often just anticipating my departure in the hour before I left would start him off. I knew this work was the best thing for both of us, so I just gritted my teeth and walked out. It was not only the money; I knew I had to start taking up a life outside caring for Kim, and Kim had to accept that. Both of us had to start letting go of each other.

Stella agreed that my work was essential. She had been worried about my emotional state when Kim was first admitted to Finchley and thought if I started getting regular work I would be able to be on more of an even keel instead of always being so frantic.

After the boost Colin Parkes gave me with the first two weeks of work I did a lot more *bona fide* shifts reporting at IRN, and while I was grateful for them I rather wondered if I was back there for good. Then a friend of mine called Mike Roberts rang me up and suggested I did some work for TV AM. Ironically I had got Mike his first shift at IRN years earlier by singing his praises to Colin Parkes, when I had no idea about his work but hoped he would live up to expectations. He did not let me down. Over the years we became close friends and he had been particularly helpful since the accident, visiting Kim, inviting us out and even having Kim to dinner one of the nights I was working.

I did not relish the idea of working for TV AM. I told him that what had happened at Diverse had undermined my confidence; I could cope with IRN because I had done it all before but television news was a challenge I did not feel up to. He assured me TV AM was so chaotic, with many people knowing less about news than I did, that it would actually bolster my confidence. I allowed myself to be persuaded and within a week was getting regular shifts. I was used to news room badinage, which I had missed at Diverse, and felt at home being back in it. I began to feel more my own person and less an adjunct of Kim. And Mike was right, the work was easy enough for me to begin to feel secure about my ability.

While Kim was at Finchley the Editor of ITN, David Nicholas, rang me to ask if we could go into ITN to see him, and Kim could also look round and meet many of his colleagues. I thought this was a good idea, it would be quite fun for Kim and was yet another experience that might jog his memory.

David Nicholas had been to the hospital to visit Kim while I was taking my two-day break in Suffolk. He had rung me beforehand to ask if he could visit and had been very kind, saying he had heard Kim was the bravest of the correspondents who had covered the Falklands war and how ironic it was that he came through that unscathed and then should have had a near fatal accident enjoying himself on holiday.

Joan Thirkettle had been there during his visit and had told me that Kim had said he knew who David was, and told him that he was head of ITV and the BBC and he would love to work for him. Joan had thought this an amazing piece of diplomacy, or maybe sheer sycophancy.

Kim felt a mixture of trepidation and excitement about the visit. He was only just beginning to believe he might have worked there; he remembered nothing about it, but one of the workers at Finchley remembered his name from the television, which both chuffed Kim and made him realise it was true. A few weeks earlier I had taken him back to IRN, which he remembered instantly, even being able to describe the layout before we got in there. He had been nervous about how he would be treated, but he made a great effort and nobody was interested in mocking him, so it went well. It gave him confidence for this more difficult and important visit.

David Nicholas was wonderful. Unlike the stereotype of a Welshman, he is terribly shy and diffident, but he made a tremendous effort to put us at our ease. He said he would like Kim to return as soon as possible, and was quite willing for ITN to complete the rehabilitation process. I said I would take him at his word, and later did, but I knew Kim was not ready for that yet. I told David that Kim should go to Rivermead first, then, keeping track of his progress, we could talk again.

David told me he was amazed at Kim's progress. Seeing the healing power of the body in those few short months since he had visited Kim was incredible. Kim had not even been able to recognise him then.

"But," I interjected, "I thought Kim knew who you were. He just gave you a slightly grander job."

David smiled and said: "He told me he recognised me from seeing me on the television. I don't think he really knew who he was talking to."

I stayed upstairs to discuss Kim's future more seriously while Kim was taken down to the news room. He was greeted by everybody and made to feel much loved. He walked out of a there a more confident, prouder person.

I tried to make Kim's life outside Finchley as full as possible, active both physically and socially. When I was not working we often went out, which Kim loved. Most of the time I could summon the extra patience needed to deal with him, going back over the conversation when he lost the thread or suggesting what he should order in restaurants. But sometimes I was so tired from working and then looking after Kim that I just longed for a normal easy conversation and would get sharp with him.

At about this time my mother returned to England for her annual three-month break over here. I told her how exhausting I was finding living with Kim, particularly in the mornings when I had to chivvy him out of bed, out of the loo and out of the shower. She gently reminded me that his morning lethargy was nothing new; the time he took to get through the bathroom in the mornings had always been a standing joke, nothing had changed. From then on I kept reminding myself of maddening habits he had had before the accident and tried not to blame everything I did not like on the brain damage. To be constructive, I set the alarm earlier so that he had time for his morning ritual, which meant we both sat down to breakfast in better moods.

One scorching Saturday Amanda had suggested we go swimming with her and her boyfriend Matthew. It was a great idea, not only did it cool us down but Kim enjoyed himself so much the other three of us had to take it in shifts swimming with him in an effort to keep up. Impressed as I was by his physical prowess I was worried about leaving him in the crowded pool alone. I started taking him swimming whenever I could after he had finished his day at Finchley. John Draper tried to help with the fitness programme by playing squash with Kim; he was thrashed in the first match and to this day has never managed to take more than two games off Kim in any session. The first evening after the match John learned the vagaries of Kim's memory as Kim kept reminding him of his defeat, and John told him he seemed to be rather selective about what he could remember. When John discovered that Kim had beaten Jon Snow at chess he went out and bought a chess set so he and Kim could play and was regularly hammered after his thrashing on the squash court. Obviously a good loser.

We would often have people round to supper in the evenings or at least drinks. Once we ran out of wine, and feeling lazy I asked Kim if he would go to the off-licence for me; I also thought it would be good for Kim's independence, but that was really a justification for my lethargy. I drew a map for him and wrote down what I wanted. At the time we were dog-sitting so I told Kim to take the dog, sure she would lead him home if he got lost.

When there was no sign of him ten minutes after he had gone I began to get slightly worried, so someone went down to the off-licence to check, but there was no sign of him. My stomach turned over and I cursed myself for being so lazy. I went to the police station to report him missing, and explain his peculiar circumstances. I questioned the prostitutes hanging around outside on the pavement, for at that time our area was full of kerb crawlers, wondering if he could have been enticed upstairs by one of them. I assured them I was not cross, just worried about his safety. They were very nice and said they thought they remembered him going by with the little black dog, but he certainly had not done any business with them. I walked to the off-licence I had sent him to and discovered it was closed, then found a wine bar where he had been, from which he had been directed to another off-licence, but could see no sign of him. I dreaded what might become of him alone on the streets of London at night. I felt physically sick with guilt, and what made it so bad was that it was all for a bottle of wine. I felt degenerate.

As I was talking to another set of prostitutes one of them suddenly pointed and said, "Look. A man with a little black dog."

There was Kim with two bottles of wine in his hands and the dog trotting along beside him. By the time he had managed to find a shop which would sell him wine he could not remember his way home. A person he had asked had misdirected him and it had taken him a long time to find someone who put him on the right track. After that I really did need a drink.

I deliberately repeated the exercise the next week. Once again he was not back when he should have been, but this time I just waited, stomach churning, determined he would do it alone, and eventually he did return.

His great escapade was when we went down to Dorset to visit my parents.

Every August my father returns home from Washington to see his five children, mother, two sisters and masses of friends during his four-week leave. I arranged to drive him to Dorset that first weekend and take Kim with me. I was so exhausted as I drove the two of them through appalling rush-hour traffic – the whole of London appeared to be heading for the south-west – that I was beastly to Kim, cutting short everything he said and being particularly impatient with him. An underlying cause of my tetchiness was that he had spent the afternoon in Queen's Square having tests and as I was waiting for him a woman died on the ward. As well as watching her die I found myself trying to comfort her husband afterwards; it had been terribly upsetting.

Swanage is a small town lying at the foot of the Purbeck peninsula. It borders the sea, and its proximity to beaches and beautiful cliff walks makes it largely dependent on the tourist trade for a living. The narrow streets are thronged with holidaymakers throughout the summer, but our house is on the other side of the hill behind a fifteen-foot hedge, which makes us oblivious of the few tourists (known as grockles by the natives) who venture up our unmade-up road to get to the downs at the end of it.

The house, set amongst terraced lawns and rockeries, is built of beautiful Purbeck stone, and a little path from it leads to the bungalow in the corner of the garden which houses my granny. It was built for her, and she has lived there ever since giving the big house over to our sprawling family in the early seventies. We only managed to live in the house properly for a year before my father took up a job in North America, where he has worked ever since despite his good intentions and my mother's yen to return home.

I have always treated my Dorset weekends as a rest cure, the thick salty air inducing much sleep, so that I would return to London rejuvenated for the unhealthy hard living there. This time was no different, and Kim also relaxed.

Both my parents liked Kim immensely and the feeling was mutual. He began to really enjoy his stay. My father decided that Kim found speaking English as difficult as most people find conversing in a foreign language, and this communication difficulty made him appear much more stupid than he was.

On the Saturday afternoon my parents disappeared for a short walk and I left Kim in the garden with an *Eagle* annual, a childhood relic which I thought might keep him amused while I went upstairs to get some sleep. When I awoke there was nobody in the house or garden so I assumed all three of them had gone off somewhere. When my parents returned from a shopping trip in the town without him we realised Kim had taken off on his own.

By this time it was late afternoon and Kim had been gone for over two hours if, as was likely, he had become bored and started exploring within minutes of my going upstairs. It was only a couple of hundred yards to the downs and from there stretched hundreds of acres of land, with steep cliffs: he could be anywhere and anything could have happened to him. Once again it was my fault.

My father pointed out that it was unlikely he was in any immediate danger. He had no sense of direction or memory of where he had come from, so he was probably lost, but he still had his senses so was unlikely to have done anything stupid like throw himself off a cliff. I agreed, but if he was lost I could not work out how he would find us again, he knew neither our telephone number nor our address and when he realised he was lost I did not know if he would ask for help or just panic.

Leaving my mother by the telephone, my father and I drove to the police station to report Kim's disappearance and explain his condition, then went up to the cliffs to alert the warden of the park there. As we described Kim to him, I pictured him in his shorts and T-shirt, with his long gangly legs and terrible scars over his knees, the shaved patch at the back of his head and his general air of wildness; he was a frightening figure. People would not help him, they would run away. And frightened people were dangerous, they could hurt him.

It was getting late and the cliffs were clearing of walkers, so my father decided to walk home across the cliffs, asking anyone he met if they had seen him.

When I reached home my mother and the car were gone, which I assumed meant good news, so I slumped down to await her return and give my churning stomach some relief. Minutes later she and Kim sauntered in through the door and my vision of him being alone on the cliffs for the night, cold, lost and unhappy, evaporated.

He had walked over five miles to a neighbouring village, Langton Matravers, and realising he was lost started asking people for help; as I had feared, many had just backed away and one had become rather abusive. He had tried to look up the number in the telephone kiosk but, typically, there was no directory. Finally he had knocked on the door of someone's house; luckily they knew of my granny and looked up our number in the phone book. They helped Kim ring my mother and plied him with tea and cakes until she arrived to fetch him.

Once again he had proved that *in extremis* he could look after himself; but I gradually began to realise his sense of direction had become annihilated in the accident. To this day it shows no signs of improvement.

Duncan had spent July holidaying in Italy with Julie, finally getting a much deserved a break. I had to keep telling myself this last bit as I faced crisis after crisis without his comfort. When they returned, they arranged to have Kim and me to supper at Julie's flat in West London.

At a first meeting it is difficult to believe Julie Christie is a world-famous actress, for she is so nervous and diffident; the confidence which comes across on the screen pays credit to her acting ability. (Duncan had told me that in order to overcome her nerves and pass her driving test she decided to play the part of someone who knew how to drive, performing so well that she easily managed the complicated manoeuvres and passed the test.) She is also one of the most beautiful women I have ever met: her screen image owes nothing to make-up and everything to an exquisite bone structure. The most lasting impression of her is one of goodness: she looks for the best in people and brings it out. Not for her any bitchy Hollywood gossip, she even makes Duncan's occasional world-weary journalistic cynicism seem nasty and unnecessary.

Her role in the film *Billy Liar* had inspired me for over a decade, helping to shape my life. She played this wonderfully strong woman juxtaposed to Billy, played by Tom Courtney, who buried himself in his dream world, afraid to take on the real one. I saw the film aged thirteen, in a Dorset comprehensive, and every time I felt myself defeated by life in the provincial backwater I found myself working in, striving to get to London, I would say to myself: I will be Julie Christie, I will be Julie Christie. The terrible alternative of ending up like Billy Liar, always dreaming of what could have been, would spur me on and make me fight the bad times. I found meeting her terribly difficult because I did not want to embarrass her by telling her how important she had been in my life, and strained to treat her as an ordinary person.

Kim did not have a lifetime of dreams to contend with but he had still been nervous of meeting her just because she was so famous. When she quietly walked into Duncan's house one evening while we were there he did not have time for nerves, and as they talked of their mutual love for Wales and she haltingly tried out a few words of Welsh on him they quickly relaxed together.

That was the past. As we drove over to dinner he became very confused. He had a faint recollection of Duncan's girlfrield Julie and he certainly remembered the actress Julie Christie but he could not understand that the two images were the same person. I hoped that seeing her would clear it up for him.

It had been a hot day and this early evening was still warm. As we pulled up outside the first-floor flat we saw Julie and Duncan sitting at a table on the balcony, obviously recalling their *al fresco* evenings in Italy. They waved graciously in Roman fashion and Duncan came downstairs to let us in.

We had a lovely evening with tales and photographs of the Italian holiday, wonderful Italian food and wine, and Kim was happy. The tremendous improvement in him since Duncan had seen him a few weeks before, when he was still in hospital, was clearly evident. Julie asked him masses of questions about his memory problems and tested his verbal ability, logic and reasoning capabilities. She did not approach it as a therapist wanting the correct answer but as a friend asking him to describe and demonstrate his problem. Her own memory is so dreadful it is a handicap to her, so she could sympathise with his problems. Afterwards she told Duncan he seemed quite normal to her.

Julie's London lodging is an enormous, beautiful bedsit. The only privacy is in the loo, which merits a room of its own. At one stage during the evening Kim went there, and when he had not returned after some time Julie became slightly concerned. I said I thought there was little that could befall him in the loo and she suddenly beamed. "Yes, I remember when you two were staying with me in Wales, he always spent hours in the loo then. What does he do in there?"

Interestingly, the evening did not solve the problem of Kim thinking of her as two different people. It was obvious from his ease of manner that he felt he was out with Duncan's girlfriend Julie. In fact, when I asked him her name he could not remember it until I prompted him in a way I often did when he was trying to name people. I asked him who Duncan was, which he managed with minimal hesitation, and then said: "Duncan and . . ." It took quite a bit of thought and effort to fill in the missing half. Having said Julie he still floundered for a while before he got her second name. However, his memory of the evening was of spending it with the famous actress and on the phone over the next few days he would tell various members of his family, still rather aghast himself, just whom he had been having dinner with.

Once when we were talking about a man we had met during our stay with Julie in Wales I tried to remind Kim how we had met him, and his response made me wonder just what his memory of her was.

"Do you remember where we met him?"

"We were with that famous person, weren't we?"

I nodded. "What's that famous person called?"

"Thora Hird," he said decisively.

Towards the end of Kim's stay at Finchley the Thames Television documentary programme, *TV Eye*, rang me up asking if they could do a programme about the delay in sending the air ambulance for Kim. I was pleased both because of the publicity against Medex and because Kim would enjoy it. The researcher and I discussed the case and possible scenes in the programme, and he thought it would be interesting to film an occupational therapy session. I knew that a few minutes from a session was the only way to demonstrate the extent of Kim's problem; however it was not my business to provide good television for them, I had to work out what was best for Kim. For twenty-four hours I tussled with my conscience and asked advice from friends; everybody seemed to think that provided it was sensitively done it would not make Kim look like a pathetic half-wit but demonstrate the terrible handicap of a severe memory problem. Sensitivity is not normally associated with television people, but I decided to take my chances, and Kim was happy to be filmed.

The filming took place over two days. On the first the rehabilitation sequences were shot, which only needed him, and on the second he was filmed playing squash and there were interviews with the two of us. I would have had difficulty being worse prepared for my interview; the evening before I had worked at IRN until eleven, then gone on to TV AM and worked overnight until 9.30 in the morning when I rushed home to drive Kim to his squash match. That evening I had to go back to IRN and do another four hours. Little wonder I looked so exhausted in the programme.

In the middle of the interview the doorbell rang. I answered it and there on the step was Jill, our courier in Lindos. *TV Eye* had flown her over without telling me. Seeing her brought back all the awful memories of the Greek hospital and as the tears started pouring down my cheeks I could hear the cameras rolling; I was grateful later that the sequence was shown without my tears.

Having watched television people operate I have a jaundiced view of them. They tend to believe the programme is paramount and all other considerations take second place, including the people providing the subject matter of the programme. They are often treated little better than performing animals and will be put through their paces repeatedly until the performance comes up to scratch.

But these people, particularly the reporter Peter Prendergast and the producer Jack Saltman, treated Kim with more respect than anyone had since the accident. The programme came at a crucial time, for as he became more aware, so he was realising just how far he was from normality. Being in front of the television cameras made him feel important; a whole television programme was being devoted to his accident, which made him feel quite proud. He savoured the two days he was a star.

We were invited to Thames to watch it being screened, and I sat and cried through the programme. We videoed it at home and my eyes still fill up whenever we show it to anyone. They had used two sequences from the rehabilitation unit, one where he was trying to get the date right, the other attempting to work out the address of the Prime Minister. They graphically illustrate his problem.

He is sitting at a table with Stella.

"What is the date?" she asks him.

"Ooh, the date," he replies. Then guessing wildly: "Is it the eighteenth?"

"No," she says. "What day of the week is it?"

"It's a Monday. . .Thursday," saying the latter more emphatically.

"Right. What month is it?"

He goes through them very fast: "January, February, March, April, May, June. . .August," he says triumphantly.

"Right."

"Oh, I got it right," he says in a surprised tone, obviously slightly nervy and showing off to the cameras just a little.

"Right. What's the date."

"Is it a Thursday?"

"The date."

"Is it the eighteenth?" He looks at his watch. "Is it the twenty-third?"

She nods.

He laughs and says: "It's unusual for my watch to be right." After a slight pause he says: "So it's the eighteenth. Is that the date?"

Stella sighs and begins again. "It's Thursday."

"Thursday," he repeats. "Is it the eighteenth?"

"No. Look at your watch."

"I have to look at it again. Oh yes, I know. It's the twenty-third, twenty-third of the eighth. January, February, March, April, May, June, July,

August," he counts on his fingers. "It's August," he announces.

"Right. What's the year?"

"1984? Is it? Or 1983?"

"Which one?"

"1983."

This was how long it took Kim to work out the date. The next sequence was even more poignant given that he was a journalist.

Stella asked him who the Prime Minister was.

"Mrs Thatcher," he replied.

"Where is she based?"

"Oh goodness, I'm remembering the road, quite a narrow road. It's not Finchley, is it?"

"Well. . ." Stella replied, not sure if he knew the constituency or was muddled because the rehabilitation centre was in Finchley.

"Victoria? It's not Victoria, is it?"

"What's her official residence?"

"Yes, I'm trying to think." He paused. "Not Baker Street?"

"No. First, what's the actual number?" He did not reply, so she added: "Is it a two-figure number or one?"

"Two."

"OK. Is it eleven?"

"No."

"Twelve?"

"No."

"It's after that, is it?"

"Well, what do you think? It's a two-figure number. Does eleven sound right? Do people say eleven or does another number sound right?"

"Ten, eleven. No – twelve, I think."

"It's ten."

"It's ten, is it? Number Ten, yes of course – Downing Street."

The response I had from people who had seen the programme assured me I was right to allow the film. It brought home Kim's condition so vividly that many women I knew, and some I have met since, were in tears. The material was handled so sensitively that his charm came through and he did not look pathetic.

The publicity led to better safeguards being set up by the travel industry itself, so I think we did some good.

The best thing to come out of the programme was meeting Tom Rayner. He had been in a terrible car accident that summer. When I saw the picture of the wreckage I could only wonder that he had survived. Like Kim he suffered brain damage from his head injury. When he saw the programme he made his wife ring me and arrange to meet Kim. He told me later he watched the rehabilitation sequences in amazement and frustration, telling his wife they were asking the wrong questions; he did not care what day it was or where the Prime Minister lived, he wanted to know what it was like to be inside Kim's head.

He had what I called a 'Cabbage Lib' approach to brain damage: he felt quite justifiably that 'normal' people (and he used the term rather scathingly) could have no idea what it was like to have brain damage and he questioned most of the rehabilitation available, which concentrated on returning people to normal rather than trying to understand and help them cope with their condition. He did not have memory problems like Kim, and all too vividly remembered being told he had brain damage. His immediate response was that the doctors had got it wrong, he was not a cabbage. His intellect and emotions were working perfectly well, but it was people's perception of what they saw on the outside, his co-ordination and communication difficulties, that defined the problem for them. He became depressed and frightened, but luckily managed to persuade his wife Sue, who instinctively knew the real Tom was in there, to get him out of hospital. She had taken him home where he could recover as he wanted. Now he wished to talk to someone who would understand what was happening, someone who was not normal and knew the problems. When he saw Kim on the television he knew this was the man.

I had come off another overnight shift at TV AM the day Tom came round, so I was sleeping upstairs for most of the visit. Tom could not have wished for better circumstances as he did not want any interpretations of what Kim was meaning, he wanted to talk to Kim; I was far too dominant to let Kim talk for himself.

There was little noticeably wrong with Tom. He still had partial paralysis of his left side which gave him a slight limp, he had an occasional stutter and spoke in a slow measured way as, like Kim, he searched for his words, but it just made him sound more thoughtful. I liked him immensely but felt his attitude inherently challenged my chosen path of rehabilitation for Kim and made me wonder if I was doing the right thing. I did not want to get into philosophical questions about brain damage, I just wanted Kim to get better. I felt Tom treated brain damage as some people regard a trip on LSD, a change of consciousness which can be learned from, an expansion of the mind. I was trying to get Kim back to normal through rehabilitation, but Tom questioned the value of normality.

Tom never actually said anything critical about what I was doing, and I have asked him about it since and he said he did not feel I was doing anything wrong; so his attitude must have awakened an underlying doubt I myself had about what I was doing. He did force me to question some of the assumptions behind rehabilitation. When one considers personality changes caused by brain damage, how much is just an understandable reaction to the condition? Surely many people would scream and shout in terror and frustration at what was going on inside their head? What amazed me about Kim was that he did not behave like that; instead he tried to be understanding about other people's reactions to his condition. I did not expect Kim to be the same person when he had recovered as he was before the accident; an experience like that would be bound to alter one's perspective on life, just as Kim had matured in the three months of the Falklands war. However, philosophy aside, I felt the most pressing need was for Kim to receive help with his memory.

Kim found Tom wonderful. For the first time since the accident he could talk to someone uninhibitedly, someone who would not think he was mad, someone who would understand. He told me later it was the first time he could say what he wanted without having to worry about the effect of his words. Unfortunately Tom lived in Norfolk, three hours' drive from us; if he had lived closer I think Kim's recovery would have been speeded up because he could work out his problems with an equal.

Chapter 8
RIVERMEAD

It was now four months since the accident. Kim looked like a normal person and for the most part acted like one. He could have a conversation and appear rational to strangers, and generally managed to find the correct word for things; he no longer called cats chickens and when he got stuck for a noun he would find a way of talking himself round it. He could now get dressed on his own and make himself tea and coffee. He could not, however, look after himself, he would forget to eat if not reminded, even if he was starving, and still had not mastered the art of cooking – although I was teaching him to fry his own breakfasts. I did not like leaving him alone in the house, but the overnight shifts I was beginning to work at TV AM made it inevitable. I would telephone him in the morning to wake him and get him up, then call him an hour later to ensure everything was under control and that he was ready to be collected by the taxi. He could carry out most tasks, provided instructions were clearly given and written down; with a map and a shopping list he could even buy food himself.

On the negative side, his memory was still appalling: he would ask me the same question about where we were going or who was coming to see us every ten minutes until I was in a screaming frenzy of frustration. He seemed totally unaware that he had asked it before.

The price I paid for his progress was the growth in him of a terrible sense of humour. In a pre-pubescent way of drawing attention to himself he would adopt appalling accents and make puns that set my teeth on edge with their crassness. He had started his accents with a few Hitler impersonations while watching a film on television about the Third Reich. I thought them quite amusing at the time. I even encouraged the Churchill speeches that he delivered, for it showed he was using his childhood memories, but like a child who has learned an amusing trick

Kim repeated his antics until I screamed at him to stop, but he was never able to resist the temptation to have one more try. It was bad enough when we were alone together but at least he would pay some attention to my entreaties to shut up, particularly since he found me an unappreciative audience. When we were with friends, however, he played to the crowd. One night when I was busy Amanda took him to an Indian restaurant with friends, and he spent the evening talking to the waiter in an Indian accent. I was mortified when I heard, and pleased that I had not been present. Luckily Amanda thought it was funny. I was certain the waiter had not found it in the least amusing.

In spite of his progress there was an enormous gulf between Kim at that time and Kim before the accident. For me his astonishing progress was not enough, my sights were set on a full recovery, nothing else would be bearable for either of us. I wanted to return to the easy days before the accident, not adjust to living with a damaged person. At times I was able to look at Kim objectively and clearly and see the gap between the reality and what I wanted for him, while at other times I acknowledged only his progress and felt certain we had almost reached our goal. At these times I felt that it was only a matter of learning to organise the jumble in his brain and it would all fall into place; just one last effort and he would be there. I fanned the hopeful embers of this latter belief to keep up my strength and resolution, for the most part successfully deluding myself. I pinned my hopes on Rivermead.

It was Monday, 5 September, when we went to the Rivermead Rehabilitation Centre in Oxford for Kim to be assessed by Barbara Wilson. The day did not have an auspicious start as both of us woke up feeling dreadful. We had had our first real row since the accident the night before – mainly my fault, of course. We had been staying the night with Kim's brother Richard, his wife Fiona and their children at their home in Amersham. I had gone to bed early because I was tired, but instead of being sensible and taking Kim with me so he had a good night's sleep before his big day, I left him watching the television. It was almost midnight when he woke me up coming to bed and I was furious that he would not now have enough sleep to do well in his tests. We started yelling at each other and became so angry that we spent an hour hurling insults at each other, then I lay awake too furious to sleep. By the next morning we were both feeling zomboid with exhaustion.

Rivermead Rehabilitation Centre is, for all its international reputation, a physically unprepossessing place; just a cluster of small tatty buildings set in a few acres of ground. I wondered what all the visiting American brain specialists thought when they came to the city of dreaming spires to look over this centre of excellence. Instead of lush surroundings and marvellous equipment they found a rather sorry, shabby setting with a few overworked and under-resourced staff in charge of the Centre's matchless reputation. To add to this sense of beleaguerment the notice-board in the waiting-room was covered with newspaper cuttings about the threat of closure hanging over the place and the valiant campaign being waged by the staff to keep it open. Rivermead is the ever-ready sacrificial lamb the Oxford Area Health Authority is willing to offer on the altar of government cuts, so the consultant has to waste time playing politics when she could be helping her patients.

Barbara Wilson appeared all that I had hoped from our telephone conversation. She was probably in her mid-forties with thick, straight, slightly greying dark hair framing her face, and dressed in quite brightly coloured clothes which were stylish while taking account of her years. She had a straightforward but gentle manner and made it clear she had no intention of fostering any vain hopes in either of us about Kim's recovery. She tried to dampen my obvious optimism, worried that I would be disappointed when my expectations were not matched.

I found the next few hours utterly depressing as Kim was unable to deal with any of the problems he had been set. As I watched him stumble through the questions, I could see that however many tricks he had developed to camouflage his memory problems in day-to-day routine life, we had been deluding ourselves that the problem was not too severe and that the progress he had made was such that with a few minor adjustments and the learning of a method of organisation, everything would be resolved.

Kim had been regularly assessed by a psychologist when he had been at Queen's Square. I had sat there twice and listened as he was made to do various tests and had been quite heartened at his achievement, particularly the second time when I could gauge his improvement as well as feel proud of his responses. However, those tests had been designed to discover what he was able to do; Barbara's found out what he was unable to do, they concentrated on his weaknesses rather than his strengths, and forced me to look more objectively at the problem. Each apparently simple exercise probed a different faculty of his memory and found it wanting.

Firstly, Barbara set three tasks which tested whether Kim could retain information over a period of time. She showed him a picture of a young woman, gave her name which he repeated and told him to remember it for she would ask him what it was later. She then set an alarm clock and told him when it went off he had to ask her when his next appointment was. Finally, she took a 10p piece from him, put it in a drawer and told him he had to ask for it back at the end of the session. Not one of these tasks did he remember.

She read him a newspaper account of a bank raid and he had to write down what he could remember. He recalled the bank raid but the details were either vague or wrong.

She made him do the equivalent of taking a message to various destinations. He had to pick up a piece of paper from the table and then go to certain parts of the room in order and touch specific items. He understood what he was supposed to be doing but again the specific instructions eluded him and he just stumbled round the room, getting it all slightly wrong.

He was shown a handful of photographs of faces, then they were shuffled with ones he had not been shown and he had to identify the ones he had already seen; he got it right just enough times to show he was not guessing, but his answers were unreliable. He did the same test with pictures of objects, with similar results.

She asked him a few basic general knowledge questions. He knew who the Prime Minister of Britain was but he told her the President of the United States was Richard Nixon – possibly indicative of where his past memory stopped.

She showed him how to punch up the date on a rather sophisticated calculator in five easy stages, but he could not quite master it, even after she had shown him a second time. Once again he had a rough idea of what he was supposed to do, but could not remember the order of the specific instructions – yet as a radio reporter he had always been able to get the best out of his cassette machine and prided himself on his technical abilities.

Finally, she gave him five pairs of words. Three of them were obviously related, like light/lamp, and two of them had no connection, such as corn/map. She read out the list to him twice, then named one of the words and he was supposed to supply the corresponding half. With difficulty he managed to get the obvious pairs, but he could not manage the unrelated words at all.

At the end of the test Barbara told us that although Kim had severe memory problems she felt she could help him and was prepared to take him for an initial four weeks from the following Monday, and probably extend it after that. Immediately my doubts disappeared as if I had not sat in the room watching Kim's memory refuse to perform for the last couple of hours. I was ecstatic and offered my thanks, saying how I was sure everything would be all right and it was just a matter of methodically organising his memory and everything would come flooding back – the problem was that at the moment he did not have a filing system.

Barbara made it clear her view was not as optimistic as mine and stressed that she would be concentrating on techniques to improve what memory he had. "I can't give him a new memory. Nothing will do that for him. What I can do is to get him to make the best use of what he has got."

She suggested Kim should carry a notebook in which he could list everything he had to remember, and proposed various tricks to help him with things like people's names, such as word association. For example, when he thought of Michael Raven he should learn to think of a big black bird and the name would follow. Other methods included using rhyming words as a mnemonic or looking for people's distinguishing features and building them into the name. However, all this was building on what was already there; she believed nothing could be done to replace what had been destroyed. I was not going to argue with her, she was the expert, but I was certain she had the key to Kim's recovery. After all, he had been making good progress with therapists who had been fumbling in the dark; here everybody knew what they were doing so he would steam ahead.

We went to the residential part of the unit so Kim could go to the loo and I could telephone Richard to arrange to meet him for lunch. Kim asked one of the nurses where the lavatory was and when she looked up to reply she said: "Didn't I see you on television last week?" (The *TV Eye* programme had been broadcast the previous Thursday.) It was the first time in his life Kim had been recognised and he was visibly pleased. After giving him directions the nurse went over to the group of patients to whom she was serving lunch and told them about the programme he had been on. She said she specifically remembered him because he looked so much like Tom Conti. A complimentary comparison, I felt.

The staff at Finchley were very pleased at the good news and Kim spent most of the rest of the week saying goodbye rather than concentrating on his therapy. There was relief as well as pleasure amongst his therapists because if Kim had not been taken on at Rivermead there were doubts as to how long he could have remained with them, particularly now that the August lull was over and there was renewed pressure for places. Few of the other people at Finchley were able to live alone, or would ever manage to be completely independent again, but Kim had me, he could be sent home. I would either have had to look after him myself or find someone who could, but he would have been my responsibility. It had been a prospect I had kept pushing to the back of my mind, because I had no idea how I would cope with it.

We had arranged to go down to Swanage and see my mother for the weekend before his admission to Rivermead. My father had already returned to the US, staying with us the night before he flew, and my mother was due to follow in the next few weeks. Rivermead telephoned just before we left to delay Kim's admission for a week. There was no point in him returning to Finchley for those days, even if it had been possible, but I wondered what to do with him for the week. His parents were moving house and although they would have been happy to have him they had enough to deal with without Kim who would have been a considerable hinderance – this was their first move in over twenty-five years. We were stopping to have supper with his sister Susan on the way down to Dorset and I asked her if she would like him to stay for a few days, but she planned to go to Bristol to help her parents.

When we arrived at Hayes, Kim was so happy and relaxed that I knew this was where he should spend his week. He remembered getting lost the last time so there was little danger of his repeating the escapade. I had only one day's work booked for the next week so I could drive up to London on Monday morning to start work at two that afternoon, stay in town overnight, then drive back the next day; for the rest of the week I too would be able to relax. My mother and Kim both agreed with the solution.

That weekend we heard on the news that an ITN camera operator, Sebastian Rich, and his soundman had been injured by flying shrapnel while filming in the Lebanon. Sebastian had been one of Kim's first visitors, and had been devastated by the sight of this emaciated zombie. His last memory of Kim had been when they working in Belfast together and used to go running every morning before breakfast. He had told his wife when he got home that he had seen a vegetable; he did not believe Kim could possibly recover.

Kim was worried about Sebastian's injuries and feeling an empathy with a fellow invalid decided to write to him. Kim's only writing to date had been his daily diary entries which were wonderfully idiosyncratic. They were normally a joint effort between the two of us as I tried to jog his memory about the incidents of the day and he wrote down his jumbled recollections. Sebastian's letter was all his own work; I did make him do a second draft as the first one was almost incomprehensible because of his convoluted way of expressing himself and frequent changes of thought mid-sentence, as well as spelling and typing errors. But the second draft was not overseen by me so the letter that was sent off was pure Kim. He even rang ITN himself to find out where to send it, and discovered Sebastian had been airlifted to a hospital in Cyprus. I included a covering letter, probably unnecessary, explaining the circumstances behind Kim's missive.

Sebastian contacted us as soon as he was home and able to receive visitors and we learned how close he had come to being killed. He had been filming in the midst of a battle outside Beirut. He was wearing a protective flak jacket to keep off stray flying shrapnel but his arms were lifted to hold the camera on his shoulder for filming, exposing a gap around his midriff where he was hit. He then endured a nightmare journey out of the war zone with his injured soundman and Brent Sadler, the reporter, as well as a soldier who urgently needed hospital treatment. The shelling continued, exploding all around their vehicle, and the driver became so frightened he kept attempting to abandon his passengers to their fate and run. Sebastian lay there in the clammy heat and darkness of the armoured truck, listening to the cries of the wounded soldier, the screams of the driver and the ominous whistle of shells as they flew through the air to land nearby, wondering if this was how he was going to die.

The Lebanese hospital where he was taken sewed up his wounds and he declared himself fit. It was only when he collapsed that evening that Brent was able to persuade him to fly to a military hospital in Cyprus. When he was opened up a second time, doctors found his wounds had not been properly cleaned and some phosphorus had been left in his intestines which had been smouldering away all the while; if it had not been found he would have died.

Sebastian told me Kim's letter had made him quite tearful, the very oddness of the expressions indicating how much effort he had put into composing it. Sebastian no longer had any doubt that Kim was going to pull himself back to ITN, if only by sheer willpower.

During his time in Dorset Kim did odd jobs for my mother around the house and garden, simple tasks that needed doing, so she was genuine in her thanks. He trimmed the hedges and built bonfires, nothing so difficult he would not be able to do it properly. Over the week she had many conversations with him and said that even in so short a time she could see an improvement. However, I could sense she felt there were only limited prospects for his recovery and that she was worried I was still fooling myself into believing eventually everything would be back to normal. She tentatively floated the idea past me a few times so that if I had wanted to discuss it I could have, but I did not want to, and, in all honesty, could not coolly assess the choices for the future.

My attitude to Kim's recovery was a mass of contradictions. On the one hand being with Kim all the time, continually anticipating his needs, helping him remember the daily things, always inserting the names, dates and crucial facts in any conversation with him, made me wonder if it was possible for improvement to be dramatic enough for him ever to be 'normal'. Then I would make myself think back to a month earlier and count up all the improvements: he now remembered his friends' names; through watching the news every day and reading the papers he had some idea of current events (in spite of his slip-up about the US President); and we were beginning to be able to have abstract conversations. Also, I was so close to him, our lives were so entwined, that the way we were living and the way he behaved sometimes appeared nearly normal. My memories of the time before were becoming more and more dreamlike, an unreal other life. Yet again, sometimes looking at Kim I could not rationally conceive how this slow, gentle person could ever regain his full intellectual capacity. How would he ever be able to take his place among the young, hungry ITN reporters? But I had to believe it to go on. Life without Kim's full recovery was too awful to contemplate. I felt that seriously considering the possibility could destroy my primitive, intuitive faith. I lived from week to week, taking pride in his improvements and telling myself firmly that as long as he continued to make progress everything was fine. There was no reason to think his progress was going to stop.

There is an immense difference between dealing with a crisis and coming to terms with a tragedy. For the moment Kim's accident was a crisis, granted a longer and more serious one than I had ever dealt with before, but it would eventually end. The belief sustained me and allowed me to go on living entirely in the present without having to face the possibility of a future spent with a man whose brain would never again function properly.

I felt my mother's worry was maternal concern that I was going to be saddled with a disabled Kim for the rest of my life when I could have found a 'better' partner. I discussed it with her later and discovered I had been unfair. She believed that however well I appeared to be managing for the moment I could not go on indefinitely. I was not the steady, patient person Kim needed to spend the rest of his life with. I might have succeeded in tempering my need for a fast, exciting life over the preceding months, but she was sure I had not eliminated my desires, only subliminated them. Peering into the future she saw me growing increasingly unhappy until there was an explosion. She said nothing to me because she was unable to offer an alternative. She could see no hope.

The night before Kim was due to start at Rivermead we both stayed again with Richard and Fiona. I thought it would be easier for Kim to be with me until he left and also I felt rather sad at the thought of only seeing him at weekends for a while. I had grown used to the routine of living with Kim and enjoyed it in spite of the effort and patience his needs demanded. A relationship only at weekends would take some adjusting to. Richard had made it clear I could stay at Amersham during the week as well, but I needed to make the best use of the time Kim was away, getting regular work now I was no longer tied to ensuring he was looked after. It also gave me a chance to indulge myself a little: I could go out alone and see my friends. I had never enjoyed just being half of a couple, but at the moment it was particularly restricting for I had to put so much effort into making Kim feel part of everything.

I had a lump in my throat as Kim was whisked away that Monday morning. Richard had done it well; Kim was too busy going through the routine of getting himself breakfasted and ready to go to have much time for either nerves or sadness. Just as he was leaving he went into a small panic about whether he had remembered everything but was quickly reassured and, before he had time to consider another delaying tactic, Richard had driven him off. I left immediately afterwards as I was working in London that day.

The first weekend he came home I felt sure Rivermead was working well. Granted I was actively looking for signs of improvement, but he did show his first indications of initiative. He told me he needed shampoo, toothpaste and other items for washing during his stay with Richard and Fiona, and insisted on going out to buy them. I drew him a map showing him how to get to the shops (literally a matter of turning two corners) and he managed it himself. He was finally taking an interest in arranging his own life. He also noticed a dud lightbulb and went out to buy a replacement. He insisted on always answering the door and the telephone, and was so friendly that anybody calling me had to chat to Kim for a few minutes first; he would happily natter to people he did not remember. I believe this was his way of showing his proprietorship of his own home, for at Richard and Fiona's he was a guest, albeit a welcome one, but a guest all the same.

Kim could now retain some information for a few days and remembered enough of the week gone by to give me a general impression. He was obviously receiving intensive but varied therapy; as well as exercises with Barbara Wilson, he would do practical things with Carrie, the occupational therapist, such as going to the shops or learning to take buses, to teach him some independence. Their efforts to structure the chaos in his mind seemed to be succeeding.

Every weekend I charted his progress, noticed the improvements and felt increasingly optimistic. One obvious signal was his method of getting home. The first Friday Richard took him back to Amersham, telephoned me to say which train he would be catching and I went to meet it at Marylebone Station. (Unfortunately the police stopped me on the way there for having an out of date tax disc so the operation was not as smooth as had been planned, but Kim had not been worried as he waited because Fiona had given him her telephone number and ours so he knew he could phone if I did not arrive imminently.) The procedure was lengthy; by the time I collected Kim the best part of Friday evening was over. So the next Friday I arranged with Richard that Kim would catch a train on his own straight from Oxford, taking a taxi to the station when the day's session was over and buying his own ticket. I would pick him up at Paddington Station. The third weekend it was difficult for me to get to Paddington, so I arranged for him to get home alone: he got off the train and took the Underground to Arsenal, which involved a change at King's Cross, then walked home. Everything was written down for him but I was still relieved to hear his key in the lock and see him saunter through the door at roughly the time I expected him. He told me it had all gone without a hitch. It was a tremendous boost to his confidence, a real achievement, not some academic exercise he could not quite see the point of, which was beginning to be a problem with many of the tasks he was set. After that he always came home alone.

At about this time he and Duncan went to watch Arsenal, as they often did when the team was playing at home. I always stayed behind; I am not a football fan, and much appreciated my quiet, solitary Saturday afternoons.

This particular Saturday Kim sat next to a friend of Duncan's, Claire, whom neither of us had met before. He told her what he knew about Arsenal, pointed out some of the players, and generally had the desultory sort of conversation one has at football matches. When they came out of the ground, which is minutes away from our house, Duncan asked Kim if he knew his way home. Kim vaguely pointed in the wrong direction, so Duncan led the way. When they reached the end of our road Duncan asked Kim the number of our house; Kim replied, wrongly again, and proceeded to walk past the house until he was called back by Duncan. As Duncan and Claire were leaving after tea she commented to no one in particular: "I can't believe these television journalists, one day Cairo, the next day Bangkok, but they don't even know where their homes are."

Duncan explained to her that Kim's ignorance was no pretentious cosmopolitanism. I loved her comment: she and Kim had chatted for almost two hours at the match and she had noticed nothing wrong. Progress indeed.

At the end of Kim's fourth week at Rivermead, Richard and his sister Susan had a meeting with Barbara Wilson to discuss progress. Richard telephoned me after the meeting, pulling me awake from sleeping off an overnight TV AM shift. His first words banished the lingerings of pleasant dreams one has on waking and shocked me into alertness. "It's bad news, I'm afraid."

He went on slowly and methodically to tell me about their meeting, describing it as dispassionately as possible, trying to pinpoint what had happened rather than convey his impressions. Barbara had told them Kim was not making sufficient progress to hold out hope for a full recovery. He was learning to make better use of the damaged memory he did have, but he was never going to get it back as it used to be. The first six months after a serious head injury was the time of greatest scope for improvement and his time was almost up. In spite of how far he had come, he still had a long way to go to get back to normal – in her estimation too far. The original injury had done too much irreparable damage, had destroyed too many brain cells, for him ever to be made new again. Barbara's aim, Richard told me, was to get the best out of what was left.

During the conversation I was glad Richard did not talk easily about his feelings, for it meant we did not have to discuss emotions, just facts. I was feeling the faintness one gets after a bang on the head or a hard knock, that sick, dizzy sensation. I could feel the rising hysteria in me and wanted to prolong this low-key conversation with Richard to keep myself in check. We went on calmly discussing the matter as if it was not the most important thing in both our lives at that moment. He told me Barbara wanted Kim to have another four weeks at Rivermead, and that he was happy to have Kim continue to stay with him for that time. He also advised me that there were various minor medical ailments Kim had developed, so it would be a good idea to take him to a doctor when he returned home that evening. He had also run out of Phenytoin, his anti-epilepsy pills, and I should arrange to get some more. We talked politely for a while longer, I thanked him for telephoning me with the news and put the receiver down.

I sat there stunned, unable to come to grips with the implications of the conversation. I thought of the improvement I had noticed every weekend and could not believe there was no hope. Was Barbara seeing the same person as I was? I vainly hoped Kim was camouflaging his ability by messing around, for if he thought something was silly, like the numerous exercises he was expected to perform, he would refuse to make an effort to do them properly. Suddenly I was filled with an unreasonable anger against Kim, like a parent with a child who has brought home a bad report card: if only he had tried harder.

This was grossly unfair and was getting me nowhere. I decided to put off thinking about what the dreadful news was going to mean and deal with the practical problems the telephone call had raised. First I had to get him some more Phenytoin.

I rang up the hospital to arrange to pick up another bottle of tablets the next morning. There then developed one of the more pointless arguments I have ever had – another example of the red tape enveloping the Health Service. The duty doctor at the hospital refused to give me any pills because Kim was no longer in the hospital. He told me to go to my GP. But as Kim had not been discharged by the hospital our doctor had no notes, and we were new in the area so Kim was not even known at the practice. I doubted we would be given the pills just on our say so. I believed the hospital was responsible for Kim until they passed on his care to our GP. We wrangled on about it, and he went to get Kim's notes. He had seemed about to give way, but when he returned to the telephone he said the tablets were stored away and could not be retrieved until Monday. I needed the pills immediately. I ended up slamming the telephone down in tears of frustration.

Still in tears I dialled Duncan's number. Fortunately for him his extension was engaged and by the time I was put through I had somewhat recovered my composure. I spoke to him about some minor business matter and then dramatically told him that Kim was never going to get better. Duncan was calm and kind but concerned enough to promise to come round and see me that evening.

When Kim returned home a few hours later I tried to behave as though I had not had that dreadful phone call. I was glad to see him and he appeared as confident as ever. Richard had told me that Kim had been in the room throughout the conversation with Barbara Wilson, even taking notes about it, but I decided that either he had forgotten those awful words or else he had not properly understood them for he seemed quite happy. He had come from Oxford all the way to the house alone again: I could not understand how such a remarkable achievement seemed to count for nothing.

We went to the doctor with a shopping list of complaints, queueing the obligatory hour. She was very understanding about the Phenytoin and said she had come across this situation frequently since a new ruling in the Health Service to lower the hospitals' drug bills had shifted the responsibility of prescribing them to the GPs.

Duncan arrived as we returned.

His visit was welcome but the conversation was somewhat strained: with Kim there we could not talk about the problem of him not getting better. I wanted to wail and be comforted and be told everything was going to be all right, but instead Duncan and I both had to make an effort to give Kim what appeared to be a normal pleasant evening. For brief moments I relaxed into myself, but most of the time I was looking at Kim and thinking: "He's never going to get better."

Duncan's presence in fact helped a great deal for I would have found an evening alone with Kim extremely difficult. I would have been so overcome by depression that I would have pulled him down with me. Being forced to keep up appearances for even that brief time set the tone for the rest of the weekend.

When Duncan left, Kim and I went upstairs to bed. I asked him what Barbara Wilson had said. He agreed that he had been in the room and had even taken down notes about it, but did not seem particularly struck by the importance of the message. I played the parent and asked him how it was going at Rivermead, whether he enjoyed it and if he was trying hard. He appeared quite happy with everything and said yes, he did try. In retrospect I think the reason he was not depressed by what Barbara had said was that she had never said anything different. Right from the beginning she had thought the damage was not going to heal and the problems were too severe to be overcome totally – she had told us both she could not provide a new memory. I had chosen to ignore her words and had not passed them on to Richard, so we both responded to Barbara's assessment now as relating to a disappointment with Kim's progress, while Kim had accepted Barbara's words and had not built up his hopes, so he felt no sense of failure.

I found the rest of the weekend terrible. We had people round and went out, so that Kim's two days in London were as enjoyable as ever, but all I really wanted to do was burst into hysterical tears.

By Sunday afternoon the strain of keeping up the false front was too much. I went to bed with terrible stomach-ache, feeling exhausted, but every time I closed my eyes to try and relax into sleep my mind was crowded with a list of items to do before Kim left that evening. They were all minor things – what I had to pack for him, what I was going to cook him for supper, what time we were going to leave to catch the train. I was winding myself up into a state of paralysis.

I explained to Kim that I could not cope with getting him ready to go, so we would make a list of things to be done and he would have to do them, I was going to stay in bed. As always, Kim was sympathetic about my sudden illness and only too willing to help. A friend of his from school, Paul Woodley, was coming round with his girlfriend Fiona in the early evening so I abdicated my responsibility to them. Knowing that someone else was looking after Kim and just being able to lie in my bed meant I could relax and begin to feel slightly better. The sharp pain was gradually replaced by a rather pleasant weakness seeping through my body – I felt too frail to think about the future, I would do that tomorrow.

My peace was shattered by Kim coming up to say he had got into a last-minute panic about whether he had packed everything, so they had not been able to leave in time to catch the train. What should he do?

My stomach seized up again and suddenly I felt swamped by Kim's dependence on me and the prospect of spending the rest of my life coping with him. I stopped myself from delivering a tirade about his never being able to get anything done because I knew that would only make him worse. I also knew that his indecision and inertia was at its highest on Sunday night because he did not want to leave. As calmly as possible I gave him Richard and Fiona's number and told him to ring them, tell them he had missed his train and would catch the next one. He went downstairs happy.

Five minutes later I realised what sort of a state I was in and how much that minor incident had upset me. I went into the bathroom and was violently sick.

Luckily the next day I had to go to work, otherwise I believe I would have kept to my bed all week, brought down by sheer nervous exhaustion.

I rang Barbara Wilson the next day, just to check that Richard had got her meaning absolutely right. I was grasping at straws. Barbara confirmed he had accurately summed up what she had said. She was kind but firm: Kim had severe problems and although he was making some progress there was no sign he would be able to overcome the consequences of his brain damage.

I thanked her and went away to think.

I spent the next two weeks trying to come to terms with the news and searching for a way of coping with the future. There were no sudden revelations and life did not stop as I tussled; some days I was only too pleased to be able to disappear into work so I could escape from it all for a few hours. I discussed the consequences of the news with no one. I gave the bare facts to a few friends but until I had come to terms with them myself I did not want to be battered by other people's opinions about what my proposed course of action should be.

If Kim was never going to get better I had to decide on the best future for the two of us. I had to find something which would work for years, not just the holding action we were involved in at the moment. Something we could both live with.

The dream that I had cherished and nurtured of a happy ending, a normal life, was shattered. There was to be no return to two independent people living together, the heated political discussions, the even balance of the relationship as we shouted or laughed together. What Kim and I were living through now was not just an unfortunate phase, it was life. This was the way things would be if we stayed together.

For, of course, unlike Kim's family, I had a choice. I could take on this Kim as my partner for life or I could walk out and choose another life.

I examined the bleak alternatives.

My only chance of a normal life was to send Kim home to his parents and behave as if he had died, start rebuilding my world without him. Superficially it would be quite easy. Most of my friends would be entirely sympathetic to my choice. Duncan would think less of me but would understand that not everybody could live up to his ideals. He would not condemn me. The few who did would just drop out of my life. Kim's family would feel justified in their earlier suspicions of me, but not surprised.

But Kim had not died, I would be choosing to abandon him. The guilt would be my shadow for the rest of my life.

If I had faded into the background after the accident, content not to be remembered by him, and allowed his family to take over as they had wanted, I would now only have a peripheral role in his life. I would be able to come and go as I pleased. But I had decided to take centre stage, take the co-starring role in this drama, told myself I was the most important person in his life and forced him to take account of me. However unconventional our relationship I was now his girlfriend. I had fostered that need in him. If I now removed myself, what substitute could he hope to find? And he had no inner resources to fall back on. I also organised his life, provided his entertainment. I arranged for his friends to come and see him, which was easy because for the most part they were friends of mine too; every weekend was packed with amusements for him. Of course those same people would visit him in Bristol, but how often? Time slips past for the busy people in London, but not for the waiting boy wondering where his friends are.

I had pulled Kim out of the childlike dream world that he had inhabited while in hospital and brought him into the real adult world with the assurance that we would go through it hand in hand. I had a responsibility for him. I could not now force him to take on an unpleasant uncertain future alone.

Staying with him was not a prospect that beckoned much more attractively than leaving. To stay was to wave goodbye to all my hopes and plans, to persuade myself that not only would I never savour the excitements I believed life had in store for me, but that I no longer wanted to. For having taken the decision I would have to make the best of it, I could not live out my life as a gesture of self-sacrifice, treating myself as a martyr.

I railed against fate for the unfairness of it all. I was only twenty-nine. Was my life now over? For that was what living with Kim for the rest of my life seemed to mean.

Every day I would have to plan for both of us, chivvying him out of bed in the morning, making sure he had all his meals, providing activity and entertainment during his waking hours, then deciding when he was going to go to bed.

From Kim I could expect love, loyalty and devotion, but I would not be able really to talk to him. His handicap was not like a physical disability where whatever help he might need we would still be able to discuss things. This bit at the very nub of our relationship. He was intellectually impaired. His lack of memory meant he had difficulty in both grasping and expressing concepts. In addition, I could not expect support or any help with any of my own problems. Apart from sex, he would not be able to give me what I required from a lover. For most of that I would have to look outside our relationship. Yet this was dangerous ground, for I could not take another lover. Kim's demands were too great to allow another such relationship to run parallel. Would I be able to bury my needs deep enough so that I would not care if they were not met? I doubted it.

What would our life be? I would be able to work, it would be a financial necessity, but I doubted if I could be a reporter. I would need a job with regular hours that would not entail me going away from home too often, the sort of job I had always turned up my nose at.

Meanwhile what would Kim do all day? The prospects did not appear good. I supposed ITN would find him some menial job, but perhaps he would find it too difficult to return and watch his friends do the work he would love to do – for he now knew he was an ITN reporter and was extremely proud of the fact. For the moment he was in rehabilitation, but that was not going to last much longer. Would he just take his place at the end of the three and a half million dole queue, and stay there, for he was not an attractive prospect for employment?

This brought up the whole question of how Kim was going to cope with the rest of his life. He was already feeling frustrated as he became increasingly aware of what he felt he should be doing but was unable to do. For the moment I was able to halt any despondency by pointing out the improvements he was making; but what happened when they stopped? I would have to find another purpose to his life; easy to postulate, difficult to put into practice. If I failed, he would just grow increasingly miserable, resenting my job and my fun as life became more and more difficult for both of us.

Among the future scenarios I could kiss goodbye was having a baby. Kim would be taking up all the energy I had, rather than being able to provide the support I would need to bring up a child. I felt this was probably the greatest sacrifice. I had coped with the miscarriage by assuring myself that in a few months I would be pregnant again – but now it seemed that had been my only opportunity. When I was younger and had appeared constitutionally unable to settle with one man for more than a few months I had managed to come to terms with the prospect of childlessness by counting the advantages of being free and single. Even my unfounded fears of infertility after I had met Kim were bearable because of the freedom a life without children would entail. But now it seemed I was to have the worst of all possible worlds, no baby, no money, no freedom.

I sat on the floor of my bedroom, my back against the wall, hugging my knees to my chest, my chin digging into them, searching desperately for a glimmer of light, for another option. In my desperation I even had fleeting visions of pushing Kim down the stairs or giving him a drug overdose.

It seemed untenable that Kim's life had been saved only to live out the next few decades in misery. It would have been kinder to have left him to die, or at least in his state of unknowing. Had he lost his protective childlike innocence only to know the depths of his own unhappiness?

But my greatest fear was for myself. However fine my intentions I felt I would betray him. Eventually I would grow so desperate I would meet my needs outside our relationship and take a lover; it seemed inevitable, whether it took months or years. Paralleling my mother's private thoughts, I knew I would not be able to live a life in which I felt trapped, in which a heavy door had been clanged shut to keep out hope and happiness. But even now I also knew a lover would not solve any problems: an understanding man would be an added complication and a demanding one could impose decisions on me.

I went on examining the possibilities from every angle, hoping that if I thought about it enough I would find a compromise solution that would go some way towards appeasing both Kim and myself, but the more I considered the alternatives, the more bleak the scenarios appeared.

I remembered someone saying to me years ago that real life was not like the movies, there were no happy endings. I had been shocked by the concept for in the innocence of my early twenties, when everything seemed possible, I could imagine nothing else. Gradually over the years I had accepted that for other people this was true, but for myself I had always counted on a happy ending – it was the way I had pulled myself through the many bad times. Now I had to grow up and realise I was not immune. There was no get-out clause from this one. I had finally been forced to join what many people consider real life, not looking for the optimum solution, just the least bad.

Still trying to work out a way forward, a strategy for dealing with the future, we went to stay with Des and his wife Pam in the wilds of Essex for Hallowe'en weekend.

I drove to Oxford to pick up Kim from Rivermead. I had finished an overnight shift that morning and caught four hours sleep before leaving home in time for my appointment with Barbara Wilson. As always she was kind but firm: there was no question of recovery. I watched Kim working at Rivermead where he seemed happy if rather less alert than at home. I was also introduced to his woodwork teacher, Mr Jones, who was a Welshman Kim had talked about a lot – the person he felt closest to in the Centre. Barbara told me that Mr Jones thought Kim was well and did not see what the difficulty was. Then she smiled at me and said that of course he did not have to deal with the problems she did.

From Rivermead we drove to see Beryl the healer. We had not visited her for some weeks, which I thought could be the reason for Kim's mass of minor ailments. As she worked on him I told her that the prognosis for him was now rather pessimistic – he had made most of the progress he was going to make. She looked rather perplexed and, holding his head between her hands, said she could feel his brain had still not completely healed. At this point nobody could say how much improvement was still to come; until the healing was completed it was impossible to say how much had been destroyed, and even then there was a lot of relearning he could do, activating previously dormant parts of his brain. Beryl was rather dubious about the emphasis on rehabilitation. She thought it could be a matter of too much too soon, comparing it to trying to walk on a broken leg. This last was said rather tentatively, but on one matter she was adamant: I was not to give up hope.

After we left her and were driving on to Des's I chewed over what she had told me: perhaps I had been too ready to trust the view of the professionals, to bow to the experts. Why should they know so much more than I did? After all, I saw Kim outside rehabilitation, I was with him when he dealt with the real world. Barbara had admitted he was still improving and had even made progress in the last two weeks. It was a muddle I knew I was going to have to sort out when I had time to think, but there was the glimmering of the possibility of another way.

That evening Des was probably in a worse state than I was. He was extremely worried about his job because the programmes he presented on LBC were under threat and the alternatives being offered to him were not tempting. The strain of the past two weeks was heightened when he got out of the crowded commuter train in the wet dark evening and discovered that his car would not start. His weekend began with a two-hour wait in the British Rail station car park at Great Dunmow until the RAC arrived and fixed it.

When he finally arrived home he poured some stiff drinks down himself before even attempting to be sociable. By the time Kim and Pam went to bed, leaving Des and me to ruminate into the small hours, he was seeing life through a melancholic haze of alcohol, and when the conversation touched on Kim he turned the black cloud on me. Not only was Kim not going to get better, he was so dependent on me that he was pulling me down with him. In fact he would probably be much better without me because he had come to rely on me so totally that together we were both going under. If anything was to survive I had to cut loose. Des was telling me to leave Kim.

I do not know whether it was sheer pig-headed perversity or the suggestion of a morally acceptable way of leaving Kim presented as the only viable option for both of us, but suddenly I knew I was not going to leave him. As I fiercely argued with Des I became aware that this was not because of some noble ideal but because I was still in love with Kim. Of course our relationship had changed, there was an inherent inequality in it and Kim could not fulfil me in the way he used to, but over the past few months I had developed a tremendous respect for the way he had dealt with his terrible problems and tried so hard not to be brought down by them or allow them to overwhelm other people. If Kim had had any idea of the agonising I had been doing over these last two weeks he would have left so as not to become a burden to me. How could I let such a man go?

To be fair to Des, he was horrified when I reminded him of the conversation a few weeks later. It had been drunken depression talking and he could remember nothing of it. However, it helped to form my resolve.

As a woman I felt there was no alternative: the reason I had chosen not to marry Kim was because I disapproved of the institution, not a lack of commitment. I had chosen him 'for richer for poorer, in sickness and in health' and I had to stick by him during the bad times.

When I returned to London I thought more about Beryl's words. She was always very careful about expressing her opinions or raising false hopes. She had been worried that Kim and I might look on her as providing the solution to his problems when she felt she might be able to achieve very little in his case; yet every visit had done him a great deal of good. Apart from curing his double vision and untrapping his nerves, there were more subtle improvements in him each time he saw her. If she said she thought there was hope for Kim, those were not words to be easily dismissed. The rest of us could only observe him but she could feel what was happening to him. If she sensed there was reason to hope, I had cause to go along with her.

For two weeks I had struggled to come to terms with Kim never getting better and had failed. No desirable, or even acceptable, scenario had been suggested to me by the professionals so I would make up my own: Kim was going to get better. I was going to live on that premise and plan the future accordingly.

The first step was to bring Kim home, for a number of reasons. Rivermead was not working as well as I had hoped. Perhaps it was just that he was getting rather institutionalised or was tired of doing abstract exercises in an artificial setting reminiscent of his schooldays and seemingly unconnected to life outside. Perhaps Beryl was right and he was being pushed too hard physically; five days a week intensive rehabilitation combined with two hours' travelling each day could be wearing him out so he was just not performing as well as he might. Possibly he was too tired to learn properly. A rest might also give him a chance to put into practice all the strategies he had been learning, to discover which he could use in his ordinary life and which were unsuitable. I remembered what Barbara had told me of what Mr Jones had said and wondered if Kim performed better in woodwork classes not just because his weaknesses were not always being shown up, but because he felt happier. He had been making a television cabinet for Richard and

Fiona in the last few weeks and perhaps this made him feel he was doing something worthwhile.

Also, I knew he minded living in someone else's house. Richard and Fiona and their children were always kind to him and made him feel welcome, but it was not his home and he felt like one of the children rather than master of his house, as he saw himself in the place he owned. I felt we needed to be at home together, to stop cramming life into the weekends so each one was so jam-packed with entertainments there was no room just to relax together. With all the other difficulties, I could see that if we carried on living separate lives during the week and only briefly meeting for weekends we would drift apart. My weekday life would be something I wrenched myself away from to spend the weekend with Kim. During the week, as well as working, which was often enjoyable and stimulating enough, I also saw my friends, and could behave as a free agent, answerable to no one. It was becoming all too pleasant. I did not want to grow to resent the weekends when I had to take up the heavy yoke of responsibility again. If Kim were at home all the time he could start developing a life independent of mine, and at the same time the focus of our lives would not be so unrelated.

Another reason I wanted Kim to come home was because I was worried that the view of the staff at Rivermead that he was not going to get better would become self-fulfilling. He would pick up their message and accept their lowered expectations of him. I knew my hope of his recovery was based on desperation and possibly a hopeless refusal to face the facts, but if there was any chance of it happening it depended on Kim believing it too. We were not dealing with a broken leg which would get better in spite of any depression on the patient's part, we were dealing with a damaged brain which made the factors relating to recovery so much more complex. I believed motivation played an enormous part. To recover, Kim had to believe it was possible.

I rang Barbara Wilson and asked if Kim could come home when his next four-week stay was over. She agreed a break would probably be good for him, he could come back to Rivermead after Christmas. However, when I told her I had decided Kim was going to get better she was concerned. I explained it was my only option, we could not continue together if he did not get back to normal – surely there must be some hope? She said he would improve, he would learn to adapt to his memory problems, but would never overcome them. She compared him to a spastic who cannot use his hands so learns to paint with his teeth, but that was all I could expect.

Having secured Kim's release from Rivermead I put part two of my plan into action. Coming home was not enough in itself, he had to do something that would give him confidence, something concrete to gauge his achievements. If he just sat around waiting for me to get home from work he would quite likely regress. Duncan and I had often talked about Kim going to work at *City Limits* before returning to ITN to get him used to doing news again, outside the high-pressure competitive atmosphere of ITN. I asked if Kim could go there when he came back from Rivermead. Duncan and I agreed on a two-week trial. If it worked, as I was sure it would, it would give Kim constructive rehabilitation and good preparation for ITN; if not, I would have to think again.

I felt that one of Kim's major problems was that while he struggled to deal with rehabilitation exercises his confidence was ebbing fast. The more Kim improved the more he became aware of the ground he had to cover to take up his old life properly, in particular his old job, and to bridge the gap between himself and his friends. He was also embarrassed to be in rehabilitation. When he was at Finchley he sometimes used to tell people who came round or phoned up that he was back at ITN. He needed to do something he considered real, something that had status and worth in his and other people's eyes. Only a job fitted the bill. I felt that going to work every day and being able to talk about his life in the office would give an enormous boost to his confidence which I was sure was the key to his progress. It was difficult to gauge what he remembered or did not remember when he was continually trying to give the answer he thought was wanted, always worried about getting it wrong. What was clear was that he made his greatest improvements when he felt happy.

All that was needed now was ITN's approval of Kim working on *City Limits*. It is a left-wing magazine and ITN prides itself on the so-called neutrality of its reporters. I was worried that ITN might have objections.

I went to see David Nicholas, the Editor of ITN, and explained to him how important I thought it was for Kim to be given this opportunity to regain his confidence as a prelude to returning to ITN. To avoid embarrassment Duncan and I had agreed Kim would not be paid, would write under a pseudonym and be kept away from any story that was controversial. David was wonderful and just asked me to thank Duncan. He understood how lucky we were to be given this opportunity.

I mentioned to Barbara Wilson that I was going to get Kim to do some work while he was in London and she made it plain she thought it would be a disastrous move. Both she and Carrie, the occupational therapist, felt he was not ready for any sort of pressure.

I decided I had to follow my own instincts; for all their expertise on brain damage and memory, I knew Kim best and, unlike them, I had to live with the consequences of my action. I knew the results of this experiment would affect the rest of my life – and Kim's.

The week after Kim left Rivermead he went to Bristol to see his parents on his own for a few days as a break before beginning at *City Limits*. He travelled down to Bristol alone and apart from almost forgetting to get off the train, until he saw his mother and his sister-in-law Little Sue waving from the platform, he was fine.

While he was there, TV AM offered me a job as a reporter. I was extremely hesitant in accepting it at first. I felt it was all right to do a few shifts there because I was desperate for the money but to take on a staff job implied some sort of commitment. Duncan, Madeleine and Jon all pressed me to take it, if only for the regular salary. In true TV AM fashion when I did accept it I was told there was no longer a job; however, after much wrangling among the management they agreed I could start on 1 January. It was quite a relief because the company's latest cash crisis had meant a ban on freelancers, which would have dried up a pleasant means of earning a living.

When Kim returned from his parents on the Thursday evening he was foul to me: everything I did or said was wrong. Finally on Saturday night it erupted into a row and when we had stopped shouting at each other I asked him what was wrong.

"I am never going to get better and you are going to leave me," he replied.

I was stunned. I asked him if his parents had told him this. He replied in the negative but said he knew that was what they thought.

In my new-found elation I had forgotten that the rest of his family still believed Barbara Wilson, they had no reason not to, and Kim was so sensitive he would have picked up that sense of hopelessness in the atmosphere.

I assured him I was not going to leave him and I was convinced he was going to get better. I reminded him that he had been virtually given up for dead both in Greece and in London but had lived, so we were just going to prove them wrong again. Jokingly I told him that he could not let me down; I had got him work at *City Limits*, then ITN were ready to take him back. He was just going to have to get better; I was counting on him.

To me it was the final proof I needed of the importance of attitude: as long as Kim was convinced there was hope he was fine, but as soon as that was removed, as had happened this week, his despair not only halted progress, it raised the spectre of the dark psychological problems we had mercifully so far escaped.

Chapter 9
CITY LIMITS

If I had had any idea of what I was asking Duncan to take on when I arranged for Kim to work at *City Limits* I do not think I would have dared request the favour; but throughout this time my blind overrating of Kim's ability made me oblivious of many of the obstacles to Kim's recovery. If I had been more clear-sighted I think I would have given up, but my determination shaped my vision.

Kim was both excited and nervous about going to *City Limits*. When he woke up on the morning he was due to start, there was no difficulty in getting him up, there was a sense of purpose and pride as he got ready to go – after all, this was his first day at work.

The old *City Limits* office was only a bus ride away from where we lived, so it was easy for Kim to go there alone. I wanted to treat him like a normal person, so I knew he should make his own way there: he was not going to kindergarten, he was going to work. That first morning I took him to the bus stop, explained what he had to say to the conductor so he was shown the right stop to get off, and gave him directions to *City Limits* from there – just a short walk down Islington's Upper Street. He quite happily got on the bus and I waved him off.

Duncan had told very few people at *City Limits* that Kim was coming, as he did not want him treated as an interesting exhibit. So when Kim arrived at the office and asked the receptionist where the news room was she directed him up there without thinking it unusual: lots of freelancers passed through the building.

In the news room with Duncan were Bea Campbell, Ferdi Dennis, and Steve Pinder the Sports Editor. They were all wonderful, immediately accepting Kim as part of the news room. They knew all about him, they had followed the story from the beginning, and they protected him from everyone else; few people knew the extent of his problems and he did not become an object of pity.

City Limits had evolved from a strike over equal pay at the other major London listings magazine, *Time Out*. The staff had always had equal pay and the owner wanted to change it so some would be paid more and some less. It became apparent after a few months that there was no possibility of a negotiated settlement, so the strikers decided to go it alone and start up their own magazine. They succeeded by paying themselves appallingly low wages and working very hard. To raise the capital for their venture they had designed a leaflet called *46 Good Reasons for Starting a New Magazine*, which had a picture of each of the forty-six founding members with short biographical details. Duncan used this leaflet to acquaint Kim with who was who. Every time anyone came into the room Kim would look them up on the leaflet to get their name, and whenever he was sent to another room to see anybody he would use it to find out what they looked like first.

That first day Duncan had managed to find a Welsh tale for Kim to work on, which was a kind effort for they do not crop up in a London listings magazine very often. Watching him do that story convinced Duncan that Kim would eventually get back to being a proper reporter, however long it took. As soon as Kim got on the phone he became authoritative and alert, he sounded like the journalist he always had been, his hard detailed questioning covering every angle of the story. Duncan said the person who was being grilled by Kim would have assumed that he was back to normal, and would have found it difficult to believe that when Kim put the phone down all his diffidence and hesitation returned as he struggled to assemble the information into a story.

He had diligently taken down all the salient points in shorthand, which had survived intact through his memory problems, but when it came to reading it back so he could write up the story he found it impossible. Before the accident he had relied on being able roughly to remember the details and his notes were just to refresh his memory, which made the shorthand easy to decipher. However, he was so overcome by nerves about doing his first story he found himself unable to remember anything relevant from the telephone conversation, and there was too much ambiguity in his shorthand for him to rely on it. He had learned there was little point in face-saving gestures so he rang the man back and made him go over the points he could not decipher again, this time taking it down in longhand.

Kim also had to ring the Welsh nationalist Dafydd Ellis Thomas and was pleased when he remembered who he was and enquired after his health, which was a good welcome back to journalism.

Kim never had to relearn how to be a journalist. From the minute he walked into the news room at *City Limits* he knew the theory of the job, the difficulty was putting it into practice. He had to learn how to adapt his techniques to deal with his memory problems, and work out ways to reduce reliance on his memory to a minimum.

It took only a few days to convince me the experiment was working. Kim's self-confidence was growing daily and while there were no leaps and bounds in his ability to remember, his growth as a person made him much easier to live with. He had begun to regain his identity and his pride in himself.

He started to use many of the tricks Barbara Wilson had taught him at Rivermead to help his memory. He always carried his notebook with him, so he could write down anything he had to remember. He had begun this at Finchley but never wrote very much in it and rarely looked at it. Now he regarded it as essential and the notebook became his memory. It worked in two ways. It held the vital information he needed, and because he knew everything was there and he did not have to struggle to remember messages he had been given, he became less fraught about his bad memory and sometimes would remember without his book. In solving some problems, it caused others: he became frantic whenever he thought he had lost his book and he often forgot to look in it. I got into the habit of reading through it to check if he had made any arrangements he had forgotten about, but the system was not foolproof.

When Kim worked at *City Limits* the office was a tip. Money had only been spent on the bare essentials, chairs, tables and typewriters, and those were tatty. There were no carpets on any of the floors, so in the news room if someone was typing while you were on the phone it was almost impossible to hear the conversation. The battered typewriters and general squalor were a far cry from the new technology of ITN, yet Kim loved it at *City Limits*. Every evening he would tell me about his day at work, happy that he had been doing something real. He never told me about the difficulty he must have had just getting through the day, pretending to be a normal person but always having to look for clues as to who a person was, whether he was supposed to know them, where anything was or what he had been told to do only five minutes earlier.

Duncan said he came to admire Kim tremendously as he daily faced the risk of being mocked or patronised if anyone realised he had no idea of where he was going or whom he was talking to. He also thought Kim showed an incredible patience with his problem. Duncan had come across brain-damaged people before, mainly through abuse of drugs or alcohol, and they were all angry at the frustration of no longer having control over their brain. Kim dealt quietly with his problem and rarely talked or complained about how awful it was.

When Kim arrived at the office in the morning he would always ask the person on reception where the news room was; it took weeks before he could get there alone and often he would have to ask two or three other people on the way because he got lost. When he reached the news room Duncan would give him something to do and Kim would diligently write down the instructions, but if he had any problems Duncan noticed that he would discreetly go over to Steve Pinder or Bea to ask what a phone number was or how to get hold of somebody. Duncan was the News Editor and as far as possible Kim tried to hide his problem from him when they were working.

For weeks he had terrible problems finding the loo. Each time he went he had to ask for directions. What amazed Duncan was that it did not seem to bother Kim that he needed help every time, he just accepted that he could not find it alone.

At least once a week Kim would decide he needed to go to the bank. So he would ask Duncan how to get there, which was fairly easy, repeat the instructions and then go down the stairs and out of the building. Duncan watched the first couple of times as Kim walked out of the office, looked up and down the street and immediately went the wrong way. He eventually found the bank by asking people in the street; it just took a long time.

One of the markers Duncan used to chart Kim's progress was his evening departure. On the first day Duncan had to take Kim to the bus stop, put him on the bus and hope that he got off at the right place. Slowly Kim learned to find the bus stop from the office on his own. At the same time he had to remember which bus he had to catch. For weeks he would always ask Duncan just as he was leaving and Duncan would tell him the numbers of the two buses. Duncan realised Kim was never going to remember the numbers alone, he needed a memory cue for them, so he and Kim devised two mnemonics: *nineteenth* nervous breakdown, and *four* Pete's sake. They were so successful that to this day Kim will reel them both off when asked which bus one has to catch to *City Limits*.

Kim had not been there long when the ITN Editor David Nicholas rang and made a lunch appointment with him. Kim knew this was important and took it very seriously. That morning he was up early, making sure he was properly dressed. At *City Limits* he and Duncan discussed how he would get there. After a few minutes' debate about tubes and buses Kim said he would take a cab because it was important he was punctual and that way he would not get lost. Afterwards Kim said the lunch went very well but he was still so keyed up he could not remember much about the conversation.

After a few days Duncan felt reporting was proving too much of a strain for Kim; just trying to function normally in a news room was a tremendous effort for him, without having to write stories as well. So Kim was given the task of constructing a filing system. It had been one of those tasks that Duncan had been meaning to hire someone to do when *City Limits* had some money, or he would do himself when he had time to spare, which of course he never did. It was perfect work for Kim: it was important without putting any pressure on him, so he could do it at his own pace and know he was being useful. Slowly and methodically he sorted it all out, and now someone is hired to keep his files up to date, so there is a lasting memento of his time there. He also acted as a news desk assistant, taking messages for all the others who spent a great deal of time out of the office. As Kim unwound in that atmosphere, Duncan, Bea, Ferdi and Steve watched him begin to blossom. He was not only gaining confidence, his memory was improving.

The experiment was working so successfully they all agreed Kim could stay there as long as necessary. So we had to decide whether he stayed there or returned to Rivermead for more therapy. One evening I gave him the alternatives, trying desperately to be objective about the choice, pointing out that staying at *City Limits* was a risk because he was out of proper rehabilitation and both Barbara Wilson and Carrie felt he needed more therapy, though I thought he would be all right without it. He said he would stay at *City Limits*.

I rang Barbara Wilson to tell her of our decision and spoke to Richard's wife Fiona to tell her Kim would not be coming to stay. Neither of them approved of the move away from Rivermead, but neither of them tried to stop it either.

I felt quite nervous after I had made the phone calls. We were now on our own, relying on friends. I had taken Kim out of the system and if I was proved wrong I expected little sympathy from those in it. Without having read a book on head injuries, brain damage or memory loss I was saying I knew more than the experts; but over the past seven months I had learned how little anybody knew. I had to weigh up my tendency always to overrate Kim's ability against the fact that I was closer to him than anybody. I just hoped I was clear-sighted enough to be doing what was truly best for him.

After a few weeks at *City Limits* Kim had an appointment to see his consultant Mr Hayward. I felt extremely tentative as we sat waiting for him to see us: I thought he was probably going to be rather angry with me for putting my opinion above medical knowledge.

He was his normal congenial self when he showed us into his consulting-room and congratulated Kim on the progress he had made since leaving hospital. I decided he probably did not know what I had done, and steeled myself to tell him while he and Kim talked. When he turned to me to see if I wanted to add anything I said I thought it would be a good idea if Kim's blood levels were checked to make sure that it was still necessary to take such a high dose of Phenytoin. I paused, took a breath and told him what Barbara Wilson had said and asked what he thought about it. He had already been told the prognosis and said that when he heard it he had been surprised, but he had not seen Kim for so many months that he thought perhaps Kim's progress had tailed off. He said the staff at Finchley had also expressed surprise because although Kim's problems had been serious he had been making great improvements there: it seemed strange that everything had stopped.

I told him it had not. I said that Kim was still improving at Rivermead but when they told me he was not going to get back to normal I had decided to take him out of there. He smiled as I told him about *City Limits* but diplomatically chose not to comment; however he told me that in his opinion I had every reason for my optimism in Kim's eventual recovery and return to ITN. We left elated.

The next day we had to go to see the ITN doctor, so that he could write a report on Kim's prognosis. The visit was even more nerve-wracking because his report could decide Kim's future: if he thought there was little chance, that was what Kim would be given. I noted that we had an even longer wait in his Harley Street rooms than we had had for our NHS consultation.

It was evident after the first few minutes of our visit that he was not going to disagree with Mr Hayward's assessment. I did not tell him about Rivermead's conclusions because I thought he should judge on what he saw, not on an opinion I was trying to prove incorrect. He told Kim that it was still early days in recovering from a head injury and he had come a long way already. He asked about Kim's memory problems and Kim said his memory retention was improving and he could easily recall events in the past few days and weeks. (I did not add that those recollections were often wrong.) However, the past was not coming back. The last ten years still consisted mostly of large gaps, so he had little idea of his personal history. The doctor told him that while the parts of his memory needed to function in day-to-day life would undoubtedly go on improving, there was no such guarantee about his past coming back. He compared it to having numb patches of skin; it was not painful, in fact people complained just because they could not feel pain there, but it was disconcerting. While much of the ten years might come back, he would probably have to live with what he termed "pools of nothingness" in his memory.

I knew I could not ask him what he was going to put in his report to ITN, but at the end I did say that I hoped he would not tell them anything which would make them feel that Kim had no future. He smiled at me and called me a battleaxe, then assured me that he was not going to write Kim off. I left happy.

When Des had been telling me to leave Kim that Hallowe'en weekend he had asked me what sort of sex life we had. I told him that as we did not see each other very much it was hardly a fair question. He said that clinched the argument that our relationship was fairly unsteady. Impetuously I decided to prove Des wrong, without thinking of the consequences, and by mid-December my pregnancy was confirmed.

I was terribly happy. I saw it as an omen, a sign of hope, a signal that our lives were beginning to get better.

There was no question of a termination, even though when I looked at my situation coldly and objectively I knew it was a leap of faith. If Kim did not get better my burden would double, like being a single parent combined with caring for someone with senile dementia. However, I was so sure Kim was going to be all right I refused to dwell on that possibility.

My pregnancy seemed a wonderful way of dealing with any weakening in my resolve to care for Kim. Going back to full-time work had begun to shift my focus outwards, away from Kim; a baby would fix it firmly back in the home. I knew that Kim needed at least another year of the security I could give him, but I was slightly worried about meeting a man who could provide an alternative attraction to the constant effort it took to be with Kim. My pregnancy wiped out any possibility of that and it gave Kim and me more time to work out an adult relationship instead of the dependent one we were forced into at the moment.

I prepared Kim for it slowly, first telling him I thought I might be pregnant, then saying I was going to have a test. When I rang him at work to tell him it was definite, his first response was a gasped: "I am going to have to learn to be responsible now, aren't I?"

I thought this supported my view that the baby might help Kim's progress; he would have to learn to look after himself as he was able to make less and less demands on me.

I had always known that when Kim began to assert his independence we would start having enormous rows, but had looked forward to it as a sign of progress. What I did not realise was that I would be an equal participant in those rows and even sometimes the instigator.

As Kim was becoming steadily more assertive I was getting more exhausted – the cumulative effect of months of looking after Kim combined with shift work I was doing and being in the early weeks of pregnancy. The combination was lethal.

One of the problems with Kim's memory was that in his efforts to fill in the gaps of his past he confused fact and fiction. Most people do this to some extent – witness, for example, the way everybody has different recollections of the same event. With him it was not so much a matter of slightly embroidering the truth as improving the flow by making up the details his memory could not supply. I am not sure whether he was even conscious of doing it. When I questioned him about it he would vehemently assert that his version was correct. Rationally I knew it was just another method of his coping and I should have let it be, but I found that course very difficult partly because I hated hearing a story that was mostly fiction and partly because I was worried he would continue to do it and people would laugh at him. Telling any fabrication that came to mind would be a hard habit to break if he started relying on it. I should probably have just let it take its course, because it was bound to get better as his memory improved.

An annoying habit that came out of it, which is still the cause of arguments today, was making up the past to prove a point: he would swear blind to never putting tea bags in the sink or leaving the oven on or whatever. In spite of his awareness of his memory problems, when he 'knew' something had happened, no rational argument would change his mind. I would end up screaming in frustration.

His dependence on me meant that everything that went wrong was my fault, nothing was his responsibility because either I had told him to do something which he should not have done, or told him not to do something that he should have done or, most frustrating of all, not told him to do something when I should have told him. If he was late for work it was my fault for not getting him up early enough, or not telling him he had to hurry; if he was hungry it was my fault for not reminding him to have breakfast, lunch or supper.

These arguments were not only a way of Kim's trying to change the balance of our relationship, at times he wanted to see how far he could push me. He always seemed to be waiting for me to say I had had enough and was leaving him. He was testing my staying power. I made sure that however angry I became during these exchanges I never lost control; a part of me understood the rational basis for the argument, so although I shouted back, hurled insults and was generally as childish as Kim, I never stormed out, threatened to leave or said something that could not be forgiven. I tried to avoid severely knocking his confidence. He knew that he did not have to behave well for me to stay and that gave him security. A real relationship was slowly and painfully beginning to evolve.

Both of us have terrible tempers that are easily aroused and we are always convinced we are right. Little wonder there were terrible rows. I would get so angry I wanted physically to harm him, and started leaving the room before he could wind me up. But Kim would never let a subject die, he would always return to it once he knew I was slightly cross and trying to forget about it. Anybody who had any illusions of me as the caring, patient woman should have seen me screaming at Kim.

As well as the all-day nausea my pregnancy had brought on, I had two bouts of bronchitis during December. My body had obviously decided it had had enough. This forced Kim to take a more active role in caring for himself and he even managed to look after me sometimes, though this was just as likely to bring on another argument. I would ask him to make me something to eat, and he would go to a great deal of effort and produce huge quantities of inedible food. Because illness makes my temper particularly short I would not be diplomatic and we would be pitched into another row.

But our life was not all screaming arguments; for much of the time we got on better than ever before because of Kim's improvement and his pride in himself.

Both of us had birthdays in December. Kim's was first and I organised a small supper party for him, inviting some of his friends and some people from the hospital. The latter were amazed at his progress: he seemed so happy, relaxed and normal.

My birthday was my thirtieth, which I had always looked upon as a milestone. When I woke up that morning I thought of all the things I had wanted to achieve and had not done, but I was not depressed. The months I had dedicated to Kim had put career goals into perspective as pleasant ephemera, but of no permanent worth. Instead of regretting the many omissions of the last decade, I looked forward to the next one. I decided this day was the turning point, the worst was over, the days in the dark tunnel when I could only feel my way were nearing an end. I could see a glimmer of light.

One copes with a long period of unhappiness by allowing oneself to believe this is normal life, forgetting what carefree happiness is. At first I had spent as much time as possible thinking and talking about the past to remind me what happiness had been like and trying to convince myself it would return. When this very painful phase had dissolved into a numbing misery and acceptance of the strange life I was leading, I had not considered myself unhappy. To me that was life and I was living it; if

I used words like nightmare it seemed grossly self-indulgent for I thought of myself as just living life less fully, not desperately unhappy.

Now I knew the worst was over because I could look back on the last few months and shudder, wondering how I had managed to remain so cheerful. I now knew how miserable I had been, only managing to survive by blocking my true feelings. To see the awfulness behind me was a wonderful freedom. It removed the unknowing effort I had been making all the time to keep up the phoney good spirits. My birthday had become a far more important milestone than if I had exceeded all my dreams: I had been given a chance to live life on my terms, an opportunity I never thought would be mine again.

So I too had a supper party to celebrate the beginning of my fourth decade and felt happily at peace, surrounded by friends and part of the laughter. Kim went out with Duncan to buy my birthday presents and came back with a beautiful antique ring, an old silk blouse and a turn of the century miniature photograph holder in the shape of a butterfly. They had even managed to dig up a photo of Kim from the files at *City Limits* to put in one of the wings; the other wing had a picture of a strange young girl from years ago, which was already in the frame.

That shopping trip with Kim is one of Duncan's fondest memories of their time together at *City Limits*. They combined it with buying Christmas presents for both their families. At first it was quite serious: Kim told Duncan he wanted to get something special for me which meant he had to go to a jewellery shop. Duncan led the way to a bric-à-brac shop and Kim chose what he wanted. Then Kim said he had no idea what to buy for anybody else, because he could not remember anything about them. Duncan took him to nearby Chapel Market, hoping that seeing all the articles on display might prompt him into choosing something. It all became slightly ridiculous as Duncan asked questions like "Does she have a camera?" and when Kim answered that he thought so, Duncan would suggest buying a photograph album. It summed up the whole farcical nature of Christmas shopping: people going out and buying presents as a duty, not knowing at all what the other person would like. The two of them were in Marks and Spencer when they started giggling. Nobody minded; they just assumed the two men were drunk.

Kim is a traditionalist and wanted to celebrate Christmas properly with lots of people. I was feeling progressively more dreadful, always nauseous, always tired, and I knew I was not going to be able to arrange the occasion he wanted. Luckily Kate and Aidan came to the rescue. They invited us over to celebrate with them. Aidan is also a traditionalist, so we had turkey, sausages, sprouts – the works. They did all the work while we just sat and watched television until the meal was ready. Kim was overjoyed at getting the Christmas he wanted, while I could just slump around in my nauseous stupor.

After the long, late lunch we drove down to see Jake Ecclestone, the Deputy General Secretary of the NUJ, and his family in South London. It was a second traditional Christmas, lots more food and even games with Jake's family. When we returned home Kim told me he felt he had had a proper Christmas.

On Boxing Day we drove down to South Wales to stay with Pat Hurley, whom Kim had worked with on the *Glamorgan Gazette* in Bridgend, and her family. I hoped that as well as a pleasant Christmas break it would also help fill in some of the blanks in Kim's memory.

His knowledge of the geography of Bridgend had certainly gone. We drove to the centre of the small market town and stopped, but he had no idea how to get to Pat's and we had to telephone her. Her husband Brian drove out to lead us home, which was only minutes away and a route Kim had walked many times. I do not know how much was to do with memory loss and how much his lack of sense of direction but it graphically illustrated the problem to Pat and Brian. Kim recognised the house and certainly remembered the people, although he was saved having to name Pat and Brian's four sons: they all had to be introduced to me and he just nodded knowingly.

All Kim's old friends always treat him as a joke and the Hurleys were no exception, in particular Brian, so it was easy to continue that relationship without appearing patronising or there being any unease. It glossed over the problems so easily that sometimes I wondered if Brian was aware of Kim's condition. It was only when he talked to me about how far there was for Kim to go that I realised what a good act Brian was putting on. The fooling around, the jokes, the continual rude remarks protected Kim when other people came round; as long as Kim could react to Brian he had a mode of operating, he could join in the fun, make awful jokes for Brian to groan at and keep people from discovering the extent of his problem.

Pat laid on a welcome home party for Kim the evening after we arrived, parading fellow workers from his days at the *Glamorgan Gazette* before him. Whatever he may have forgotten of the streets of Bridgend he certainly remembered the people and was overjoyed to see them again. Realising how many of them cared about him built up his confidence and it was an easy gathering, with people reminiscing about the days when he was a local cub reporter. The men stood around in the kitchen with their drinks (while we women sat around a table) and had the sort of male conversation it is very easy to be part of without much effort, just requiring the odd exclamation every now and again.

On the way down the car's gear box had jammed and the garage in Bridgend said it needed a new one. It was Christmas week and we were miles from a major town so day after day when we rang the garage they told us they had not managed to locate a new one and we had to extend our stay with Pat. I felt terribly guilty because as well as looking after her husband and four sons, her mother was also staying. On New Year's Eve it was apparent the car would not be ready until the middle of the next week. As my first day at work with TV AM was 1 January, I had to leave Kim with Pat so that he could drive the car home, and early on New Year's morning I crept out of a sleeping house to catch the train back to London.

The great problem with my TV AM job was telling the management that I was pregnant. I knew I had to do it but wilted at the thought of the anger it would cause. I had taken the job before I knew I was pregnant; I had had a slight suspicion but I did not voice it because my experience at Diverse had shown me just how willing a management is to kick a woman when she's down.

On my first day I decided to tell Sue Inglish, the union representative, or Mother of the Chapel as we call them in the NUJ. I wanted her forewarned in case she had to do some heavy negotiating for me. She roared with laughter at the news, gloating over the horrified reactions she anticipated from the TV AM management with whom she had had so many confrontations she was pleased at the thought of them squirming. Good as it was to have her on my side, it hardly lessened my nerves about breaking the news to the bosses.

The next morning I awoke with blood on my sheets. My stomach turned over. Surely I had been through enough, without having to cope with a second miscarriage? I went to the doctor who advised rest and told me that if the foetus was going to miscarry it would, and there was nothing I could do to stop it. I returned home, rang TV AM to tell them I would not be in until the next week and then rang Duncan to tell him Kim would not be back at *City Limits* until after the weekend. I managed a perfectly calm conversation until he said he wanted to get hold of me later in the week and asked if I would be at work.

I burst out: "I'm not at work all this week. I'm off sick. I'm in the middle of a threatened miscarriage. Duncan, it's just not fair. It's 1984 now, everything is supposed to be all right this year. All the horrible things should be over."

Poor Duncan was immediately landed with coming round that evening to cheer me up, not too difficult a job as I was feeling quite fatalistic. I was stonily calm, barely allowing myself to speculate. I just had to sit and wait for the outcome. The last few months had taught me to conserve my energy for the fights that mattered, the ones I could win. I knew I had no control over this one.

I told Kim on the phone, but I don't know how much he understood because I was careful to underplay it and his gynaecological knowledge has always been sparse. I certainly did not think it warranted him returning to London, because there was nothing he could do and it would just worry him.

Before Christmas I had arranged to see a friend of mine in Brighton and went down a few days earlier than planned. Carole Bentley and I had worked together in the news room of BBC External Services during my six-month contract there in 1978/9 and had seen each other more and more infrequently since. She had written to me after reading of the accident in the *Sunday Mirror* and I had invited her to my birthday do, but she had been working in her new job as Foreign Duty Editor for BBC Radio News. Carole was wonderful. We had a lovely few days together, with me glorying in being allowed to play the invalid.

By the weekend I was still bleeding slightly but decided I had given the foetus long enough to make up its mind whether to go or not, so returned to work on the Sunday. That was also the day Kim was returning to London. I had decided it was easier for me and better for him if he drove alone. Bridgend to London is not as difficult a task as it might appear because the first 200 miles are just straight down the M4; I was slightly worried about him navigating London, but Brian Hurley wrote down step-by-step directions from a road map. If he did get lost he could always ring me at TV AM for directions.

My real worry was Kim speeding on the motorway. The accident had done nothing to temper his driving which has always been fast and aggressive. We had spent much of the journey down to Wales arguing about his speed; he still thought 110 miles an hour was reasonable for cruising, while it terrified me. The accident had cured me of my adolescent love of speed and excitement and I would never rid myself of the guilt of not asking Kim to slow down before it happened, although I had known we were going too fast. On the Sunday morning I rang him up and made him promise not to exceed 80mph, a reasonable compromise, I felt, as I knew he would not agree to keep to the speed limit. I did not think it would have much effect, but it was all I could do.

I need not have worried, there was no accident and Kim even managed to traverse central London with barely a wrong turn. He told me that every time he looked at the speedometer and saw it rising he could hear my voice telling him not to go above eighty and immediately slowed down. I did not quite believe I had been so effective but I had probably stopped him from speeding too outrageously.

Kim had had a wonderful week in Wales without me. When Pat had returned to work after the Christmas break she had taken him in with her and he had gone out reporting. At the council meeting he found everybody remembered him, had read about his accident and congratulated him on his recovery.

Pat wrote a piece for the *Gazette* about his remarkable progress and the Cardiff paper rang him up to interview him. A piece appeared the next day. He showed me the cuttings, which were on the whole quite funny. In each one was a story about the Falklands with Kim's normal lack of attention to the facts. I told him that in future he should get journalists to check their stories with me because he could end up libelling someone: if the article had appeared in a national paper it would have led to a letter of apology at least.

In one of the articles Kim was talking about getting better and said that he did not believe he would ever be well enough to return to his old job. He had never said this to me. I was upset both because he really did think he would never get back to normal again and because he had had to carry this nagging doubt secretly. I had been such a tyrant he had not confided in me and I had had to read a newspaper article to find out what he really thought. I talked to him about it and he told me he did not always think that way but he felt he had so far to go before he was back to normal, at times it seemed impossible that he would ever get there. He said he had fixed his goal as going back to ITN and being a reporter, but the closer he got to it the more impossible it appeared that he would ever reach it.

The next week as I waited for my antenatal appointment to discover if I was still pregnant I buried myself in work, desperately trying not to think about it. I had finally stopped bleeding but I knew this meant nothing. When I went to my appointment the senior registrar, Mr Marresh, said he thought I was all right, but he arranged for me to have a scan to be certain. When I arrived for my scan the next day I was seen by the same woman who had dealt with me the last time. She remembered me and was extremely sympathetic when I told her I was here once again to find out if the foetus was dead or alive. She was very happy to be able to point out the beating heart and a wave of relief swept over me. For the first time I knew how tense I had been, how the calm I thought I had been feeling had been a rigidly imposed safety mechanism to stop panic. It was so good to know there was going to be a baby. The radiologist gave me a picture of the scan, the tiny curled up foetus barely distinguishable from the rest of the sac in the womb.

The next week I went into work and told my immediate superiors, the men who had hired me, Clive Jones and Peter McHugh. They took it well, Peter even genuinely congratulated me. The man I dreaded facing was Greg Dyke, the Programme Controller.

When I was still a freelance we had had a slight altercation. Not knowing who he was I had sharply sworn at him because he was getting on my nerves, jumping up and down complaining about our coverage of the discovery of Cecil Parkinson's affair with Sarah Keays and her pregnancy. To his credit he had only looked surprised and had not had me thrown out of the building; I was only told who he was when he had gone away.

I knew Greg had opposed my appointment, though I was assured it was not personal, he had just decided to put a blanket ban on hiring. It had taken Peter and Clive two hours to change his mind. Greg's loathing of middle-class women was also well known, so all of that, combined with my pregnancy, was going to leave him furious.

Worse was to come. The next week Sue Inglish stood down as Mother of the Chapel and no one was prepared to take her place. Since I was a member of the Broadcasting Industrial Council, the union body which deals with all broadcasting matters nationally, I could not allow the chapel I was in just to fall apart, whatever my personal predicament. I said I would do the job for three months, which gave them time to find someone else.

I had been on the Broadcasting Industrial Council since TV AM had started and it had rarely been off the agenda as it faced crisis after crisis, so I knew it was not going to be an easy job. However, I did not expect to be told a few days later that the company wanted twenty NUJ redundancies.

I spent the day they were announced in a series of meetings with various tiers of management and learned how much of negotiating was just macho posturing. I was shouted at by the Chairman Tim Aitken in the morning, had a chapel meeting over lunchtime, and exchanged veiled threats with Greg, Clive and Peter in the early afternoon. By the time we were due to see Tim Aitken again I was feeling utterly drained. As we were waiting outside the Chairman's office, Greg bounced up to me, looking exactly like an animated garden gnome, short with a bald patch topping his blond hair and beard. "I hear congratulations are in order," he said. "We are going to have our first TV AM baby."

He was delighted and with that worry lifted I felt I could put up with anything, even Tim Aitken shouting at me again.

At *City Limits* Kim was back doing stories, and still steadily gaining in confidence. I did not realise how much until we were visiting Jon and Madeleine one evening and he talked about going to a press conference on getting British people in foreign prisons transferred to do their time over here. Jon rather glibly said he could think of rather more important causes to get worked up about than drug smugglers who had got caught. Kim quietly and steadily explained what the conditions were in many of the prisons and the swingeing sentences many people were serving. He convinced us all it was a worthy cause. I was amazed at how easily he had been able to summon up his arguments and his retention of all the salient facts.

David Nicholas had agreed that Kim should return to ITN on 1 February and he was getting into a terrible state about it: wanting desperately to do it but dreading it all the same. He was worried he would not be able to cope and had started having problems sleeping because of all his worries. Bea and Duncan both felt he should stay at *City Limits* longer, a month or two, so he would start off from a much more confident base. I felt that as ITN had already become an issue, and all he could think about was whether he would be able to manage there, he should return and get it over with.

I was wrong and they were right. If he had stayed at *City Limits* a few weeks or months longer the worst of his memory problems would have disappeared before he returned to ITN. But my impatience combined with my refusal to acknowledge the extent of Kim's problem meant I made the wrong decision and he returned to ITN too early.

There is no doubt that Kim would never have been able to cope with ITN at all without those months at *City Limits* and he will always remember the friendship he was given there. Duncan says we should not be grateful to the people in the news room for all that they did for Kim. He says the current climate does not encourage people to help anyone except themselves, yet most people welcome the opportunity to do so. It is much harder work being helped than helping someone else.

Chapter 10
ITN

Kim's first day back at ITN was quite spectacular. It began with a live interview on TV AM about his miraculous recovery. I had not instigated this, it had been Peter McHugh's idea. He had told his wife about Kim and me and she said it sounded much more interesting than most of the items she saw on *Good Morning Britain*, and so the idea was born. I was quite willing to go along with it and knew Kim would enjoy it, but did not want to work on it because I had no professional detachment, though I did suggest they showed excerpts from the *TV Eye* film, when he did not know where the Prime Minister lived and could not remember the date, to demonstrate the scale of the recovery.

Unfortunately the item misfired. Due to some cock-up, the presenter John Stapleton talked over the *TV Eye* pieces, so unless one remembered the documentary it was difficult to understand why the sequence was used. In the actual interview there was this apparently normal person trying to convey how bad his memory had been by telling some of the stories I had told him of the intervening months. Not only was the trauma of the last ten months lost, the problems he was still encountering were completely hidden. Kim could easily deal with a five-minute live television interview, an experience most people would find a gruelling ordeal, yet he could not manage many simple things in life. His memory was still so bad he could not be relied on to remember anything unless it was written down. He still asked me directions if he was going to the shops, and for anywhere further afield I had to draw him a map. He was aware of the limitations of his memory and the effect it had on his social persona. He thought people did not like him for himself and just pitied him, so he felt inferior to everybody. John Draper was helping this immensely by still coming round to be thrashed at squash and chess every week, yet Kim always felt he was running just to keep up with people and he still tried to give them the answers he thought they wanted because he had no confidence in the ones he wanted to give.

At the end of the interview John Stapleton congratulated Kim on approaching fatherhood. Luckily we had already alerted our immediate families, but a lot of other people we knew found out about it that morning.

Afterwards Kim was rushed off in a taxi to ITN, where he was overwhelmed by the reception. Everyone wanted to congratulate him on coming through and welcome him back to the fold. He spent the day just wandering around talking to people. He returned home that night extremely proud. With that first day over we thought he had managed to conquer the most difficult hurdle; neither of us had any idea of the patience and resilience he would need in the coming months, which were to be the toughest yet.

At first Kim did only a three-day week, for both David Nicholas and I felt any more would tire him, however little work he was doing. Just trying to learn where everything was and who everybody was, combined with the atmosphere of buzz and excitement, would be exhausting.

Everybody at ITN was pleased to see him back, and those who had visited him in hospital were amazed at the progress he had made. But nobody thought he would ever return to being a reporter again. He was much better, but he could not even find his way around the building or remember anybody's name, so how could he possibly make a television reporter?

At first nobody knew quite how to deal with him. They were all rather embarrassed by his handicap and not sure whether they should pretend he did not have a problem and ignore his difficulty or try to help him. Kim resolved the quandary by being quite frank about the tiny amount he could not remember and it became an easy joke.

He did struggle to camouflage the extent of his problems. He would wander around the building when he got lost, desperately looking for clues to where he was going. He would also try to cover up not knowing who anybody was by greeting everybody effusively as if he remembered them.

After a few days Sebastian Rich, the camera operator hurt in Beirut, decided Kim was just sitting around wasting his time. It was during the English lamb dispute, when French farmers were picketing English lorries, and Sebastian was being sent to Dover to cover the story with reporter John Suchet. Sebastian suggested taking Kim, and ITN agreed. It was a wonderful idea.

They picked him up on Saturday afternoon and what was meant to be twenty-four hours of monitoring Channel ports turned into a few days in Paris doing a completely different story. Not a single frame of what was shot appeared on ITN, but that was not Kim's problem. For the first time in almost a year he was on an ITN story and he was abroad. For those days he was very happy.

While he was away, David Nicholas and I talked about what Kim should do and I suggested the Sports Desk. It was small, and if he was allowed to do more than fetch tea and coffee or answer the phone he would enjoy it and do it well because it was a subject that interested him.

The Sports Editor Mervyn Hall responded with great humour. He consciously decided to turn Kim's memory problem into a joke and was always telling stories about Kim's dilemmas and teasing him about it. When they were in restaurants he would pull Kim's leg about having forgotten what he had ordered. The stories he told about Kim being sent out of the office on an errand and getting lost and having to phone Mervyn to ask him how to get back to ITN were legion, and very funny. It sounds cruel but it was a way of showing acceptance and right from the beginning Kim had been prepared to have people laugh at his condition. Laughter was a lot easier to swallow than pity.

At TV AM I was becoming increasingly exhausted. The redundancy fight was tiring. I knew the management were not joking when they talked about a cash crisis, but I had a strong feeling my members were not in the firing line: the company managers were after the technical staff as they wanted drastic rosta changes which would save a lot of money. The attack on us was just a foil to make the ACTT believe they were not being picked on. Redundancy numbers are always negotiable and Greg already had about twelve vacancies on paper through unfilled positions (which explained why he did not want to hire me); he was not intending to ask anyone to leave. My problem was persuading people to stand firm and stay. For the many unhappy people there, the opportunity of being paid to go seemed too good to miss and for the other frightened people letting other people go meant their jobs were safe. I had to instruct nobody to leave for ten days.

The management were also refusing to guarantee we would be paid that month. I felt this was immoral, but my suggestion of a withdrawal of good will in the form of an overtime ban was rejected. TV AM became an increasingly unhappy place to work as people showed their anger in more subtle ways and became increasingly bitter and worried. I seemed always to be either in meetings myself or waiting for the outcome of other people's as the company desperately trawled for more cash and all our futures hung in the balance. As Mother of the Chapel I felt responsible for all these people and worried about how many of them would fare if TV AM did go under.

I felt I had a strange role. I had only just started there and everybody knew that in a few months I would be leaving to have my baby. Yet at no stage was I accused of being an outside agitator: not when I lost my temper with Peter McHugh and abused him so much he ran out of the building to escape my insults; not on the many occasions that Tim Aitken bellowed at me, stabbing his finger at me as he shouted that "you guys just have no idea" (in fact Aitken did get milder with me as my pregnancy became increasingly apparent, showing there was some finer feeling underneath that Neanderthal exterior); not in the crusty exchanges between Clive Jones and myself. Even the chapel accepted that I had their best interests at heart. To repay the faith I did my best, but it could only be a damage limitation exercise as we were buffeted by the continual winds and storm of management.

After four weeks we had guaranteed salaries, a surviving company and nobody had lost their job but I was pale green from exhaustion. I was due to go filming up north but Peter McHugh ordered me to take a week's rest.

Kim was having to get used to not being top priority rather sooner than expected, but I was too busy trying to sort out the TV AM mess to feel guilty about it. He still told me about his day every evening. He was not being stretched on the Sports Desk, but was enjoying himself and was pleased for just having managed to get back to ITN. His growing confidence made him tolerant of the toll union duties were taking of me, both the hours I was away from home and the state I was in when I returned – able to do nothing but flop in front of the television.

On Valentine's Day he shamed me by producing a card as I woke up. I had not felt up to the effort of buying one, being sure he would not remember; so I made a quick dash to the shops at lunchtime to have something ready when he came home.

As soon as the worst of the union business at TV AM was over I had to do some filming which took me round the country; then I was a delegate to the Women's TUC Congress in Torquay.

At that time the congresses were held in various seaside towns, always in mid-March, so the walk to and from the conference centre was in spring gales. The year before, in Scarborough, I had been pregnant – those were the days before everything went wrong – and it was strange to be among the same people and pregnant again. The conference was, as always, fun, with our delegation fulfilling its traditional role of trying to change the structure so it became more powerful instead of being a sop handed to the little ladies by the men of the TUC. Our attempts normally failed, but by smaller and smaller margins.

When I arrived home afterwards, exhausted by the hustle and bustle, the lack of sleep and long train journeys, the house was empty. Kim did not return that evening and I could find no message giving a clue to his whereabouts.

The next morning Ian Edwards, an ITN sports reporter, rang to sort out with Kim what time they were going to meet at Twickenham to see the England-Wales rugby international that afternoon. I knew nothing about the arrangement and had to admit he had temporarily gone missing, but promised I would try to find him as soon as possible. The international was far too important to Kim to just leave him to come to his senses wherever he might be, too late to be able to get to it.

I knew he had been to Birmingham while I had been away and decided to start the hunt there. I made a series of embarrassing telephone calls, including one to BRMB, the local commercial radio station, where I knew Kim had been. Eventually I came up trumps by calling the parents of Andrew Burn in Stratford and found him there. I was so pleased with my detective work I did not particularly berate him for not leaving any hint of his whereabouts, and he managed to get to the rugby to see Wales win. Ian Edwards found it a colossal joke.

At about this time Kim started going to see a psychologist who specialised in people with head injuries.

When I saw Kim the evening of the first appointment he was very pleased with himself. His interview had gone well, he liked the psychologist immensely and had been told he was making remarkable progress. He had done a series of tests on a computer which probed various functions of his brain. The results were given in percentiles, so it was not merely a matter of how many he got right or wrong but where he stood in relation to the rest of the population. On most of the tests he was scoring average marks, which was good news indeed for it meant he had the same intellectual capacity as many 'normal' people. The psychologist pointed out that one would expect someone of Kim's educational achievement to be in the top ten per cent, but there was lots of time for improvement. For the moment Kim felt proud of being normal. His appointment gave him a confidence that carried through for days. I promised to accompany him to his next appointment in six weeks' time.

In the four months since returning to ITN Kim had progressed enormously. He was no longer the rather vacant person who was not sure where anything was or whom he was speaking to. He had been taken off the Sports Desk and made to do 'real work' in what was called the production unit. It was during the miners' strike and Kim had to make daily check calls to the pits and the union to find out how many people were crossing picket lines and the extent to which coal production was being affected. He hated desk work and would have much rather been out reporting, but it was a start.

The man who had found Oxford Circus underground station a meaningless maze during his first week back now treated his journeys to and from work as routine. He was no longer challenged by work, but his frustration was necessary for him to move himself on. He still had memory problems, so that if he lost concentration he could completely forget what he was meant to be doing, but he no longer found himself always running just to keep up at ITN.

A week before I gave up work Kim was asked to go to Wales to do a background piece about the miners linked to interviews with men who had taken redundancy at nearby Llanwern steelworks. He was overjoyed. Finally he was going to do a proper story. They sent someone to help him, but he was still out doing what he wanted to do.

Aidan came round to supper the night the programme went out and we all watched it. The piece was only two minutes long, but I thought it was great, with a tightly written script and good pictures. It showed the plight of the miners and underlined their cause when a former Llanwern steelman strongly expressed his regrets at taking redundancy and advised the miners not to follow suit. I was glad to see Kim had not lost his touch.

The news desk rang up to congratulate him, and phoned again later to say they had taken calls from people saying how good it was to know Kim was back again after his accident. Then the man who sent him to Wales rang to say thank you.

I had hoped that now he had proved he could do it, the worst would be over, but in many ways it had just begun. Kim had had a taste of what it was like being back doing the job, and he wanted more, but now he had to start seriously working towards it.

He did. He asked if he could come off the production unit and start shadowing reporters, so he could relearn all the techniques. This rather put the news desk on the spot. Nobody knew how long this could go on or what was going to happen to Kim eventually, but they complied with his request and sent him on stories where he could learn and also be helpful. As long as he was keeping himself occupied and apparently happy it kept the problem at bay, though his push to get back as a reporter was sooner or later going to raise the thorny question of whether it was a viable possibility.

When Woman Police Constable Yvonne Roberts was killed outside the Libyan Embassy, which led to the ten-day seige, ITN mounted a major operation to cover it. Kim went down there to be what help he could, mainly taking messages, and spent many days watching it all. Then ITN sent Terry Lloyd to Libya to cover the story from there.

Terry had been doing freelance shifts at ITN when Kim first joined the staff and had been hired when a vacancy came up. They were contemporaries and had expected to get the same calibre story – until the accident. Seeing Terry on the television reporting from Tripoli suddenly made Kim aware of what he was missing. If there had been no accident it could have been him who was sent; instead he was in London, a behind-the-scenes minion.

It was a turning point. The depression I had been half expecting for months finally set in and he started moaning that he was never going to get anywhere because of the accident, he would never be any good, no one would ever give him a chance. This mood persisted for much of the next eighteen months. I was grateful it had begun so late, or else he could never have made the tremendous progress he had so far managed.

I knew that however painful the situation was for him, wallowing in self-pity was not going to achieve anything. If he was to return to his place as a reporter he would have to earn it; that was going to take hard work but it would be worth it. To begin with, I suggested he increased his workload to four days a week. This was not the sort of sympathy he wanted. He told me he could not cope with more than three days a week and keep up his social life, and the latter was very important to his recovery. I knew he was not completely physically fit but I sternly pointed out that I was almost seven months pregnant, large and uncomfortable, and I managed a four-day week on top of union negotiations and arranging and partaking in his social life; I thought he had rather a weak case. We agreed to leave it until his next visit to the psychologist later that week when I would accompany him.

The psychologist was a dark, good-looking man probably in his late thirties. I noticed his monogrammed shirt and his tie with the Harrods label and assumed there was quite a lot of money behind him. He sent Kim into another room to do more tests on the computer and then spoke to me privately.

He began by telling me that according to all the medical evidence Kim should be lying in some small, dark, forgotten ward of a big hospital or mental home, with us dutifully but hopelessly going to visit him, although he would neither recognise us nor communicate; instead we were talking about someone who was back at work, albeit with the indulgence of ITN, and living a fairly normal life.

He understood that being told how lucky Kim and I were did not make the problems we were facing any less and it was not good enough just to be told to be grateful for the progress Kim had made. He told me the tests suggested that the brain damage from the accident was minimal; most of the difficulties Kim was facing were from post-accident trauma. He explained that what Kim had experienced in the immediate months after the accident would have been terrifying. He woke up to find he did not know what had happened, where he was, who he or anybody else was, and on top of that was unable to communicate. At one blow the social crutches he had built up over a lifetime had been removed. This could take years to recover from; what was surprising was that he was so sane. The psychologist stressed that Kim's self-confidence had taken a terrible blow and he needed to learn to trust again.

This brought us into the area of our relationship. I found it extremely difficult to talk about it partly because I was not sure myself. I did emphasise that I knew couples who were going through much more difficult times than us, without the stress we were coping with. There was a genuine fondness and mutual respect between us which was lacking in many other relationships. However, there were certainly problems. The greatest was Kim's continuing dependence on me. It was dragging both of us down. Somehow Kim had to become more independent. The psychologist agreed but warned me not to be in too much of a hurry. Kim was taking on a lot of challenges at the moment and had to deal with ITN alone; he still needed me to fall back on, a reliable source of cheer and sympathy to come home to.

When he asked me about specific problems I told him Kim was hypersensitive when anything went wrong. If he forgot his wallet or his diary he would just collapse and tell me that his memory was appalling and he was never going to get better. I found this particularly difficult as my life burbled on in disorganised chaos with my belongings strewn among the many places I visited. If I worried every time I left a wallet, coat or handbag anywhere I would be a gibbering wreck by now. The psychologist was more sympathetic to Kim's reaction, as he also worried when he forgot anything, but he did agree that Kim had to learn to be more relaxed about it.

Most of my complaints were on that petty level, but a catalogue of apparently minor grievances can become an intolerable burden. For instance Kim would never organise his social life, expecting me to do it and then he would forget who was coming round. The psychologist said he thought this was a normal male thing.

I told him about the shopping. I hate shopping and as I grew increasingly large had been trying to shift the burden onto Kim. On Good Friday a schoolfriend of mine who lived in York and I rarely saw came to see me. To give us time to chat on our own I sent Kim to the supermarket to buy some lunch. Two hours later he returned having spent almost £50 on things he thought might be useful. I restrained my temper and only said I thought he had been rather excessive. The very next weekend the same thing happened. He managed to spend over £50 this time. I was furious. He had bought so much frozen food it would not all fit in the freezer, so it was just going to melt or go off. What made me really angry was not the expense, although that was difficult enough to swallow, but that I could not trust Kim to go shopping on his own and in my great floundering whale-like state would have to continue to drag myself up and down the aisles of Safeways. I admitted to the psychologist that Kim was known for his excesses in supermarkets before I met him and was again told that this was a male thing rather than just a result of the accident.

He asked me once more about our relationship and I felt quite defensive about it. Of course it was not normal, and there was not the sort of equilibrium I would have liked, but it was getting better. I felt I was rather oppressive, but had learned that if I did not organise everything and tell Kim what to do, nothing would ever get done. However, my work and union commitments meant he was spending time on his own and learning to do things alone, though not all of them were particularly constructive. One day I was stuck in hours and hours of negotiations and had rung home to say I would be late. Kim assured me he was quite all right, he had just been putting weedkiller on the dandelions on the lawn. I had spent the last month working hard on the garden and went apoplectic because I just knew he had ruined the lawn. He could not understand why I was so furious because he thought it would kill only the dandelions and he hung up on me. During the next adjournment I rang him back and apologised. I managed to massage his feelings, but the lawn was lost and over the next few weeks I had to watch it die.

I thought our relationship would improve with Kim's progress, which was particularly linked to his progress at ITN. His confidence would grow as he became more sure of himself at work and so the balance would even out between us. The other factor in our favour was the baby. Kim had always been good with children; looking after his own child and having someone who adored him unquestioningly would do him a great deal of good.

Then Kim came into the room to say he had finished his tests. The psychologist went to get the results and was surprised at the improvement. They were still not the results one would expect from somebody of Kim's intelligence, but he was now above average. Still to be improving at this stage was an achievement in itself, but to be improving from such a high level was good news indeed.

When we left I told Kim the results made one thing certain, he was ready for a four-day week. He knew when he was beaten and accepted it.

At the end of May I left TV AM to wait for the baby to arrive. The last week was dreadful. Not only was I enormous and exhausted but Greg Dyke resigned. My many negotiations with him had altered my view of him as a Napoleonesque ogre to liking him tremendously. Over union matters we would always clash, but those were our roles in the company. Personally and professionally I had a high regard for him. I was glad to be getting out as I knew the immediate weeks after his departure would be uncertain and unpleasant as the ambitious jockeyed for position. The last few days of my term at TV AM were full of hysterical turmoil which took their toll. I had to spend most of the next week in bed.

About a month later I realised Kim and I had not had a major row since I had left TV AM; it showed me how impatient and intolerant my exhaustion had made me.

The weeks before the birth were very peaceful: I was enormous and could move only slowly, there were no demands from TV AM, no union negotiations, and I could relax. We started going out more and entertaining: I was again providing the sort of support system Kim enjoyed.

Work gradually got better for Kim. He no longer went out with other reporters but started doing stories alone, though they were always simple and tended to be unimportant, which meant they were often dropped from the bulletin. Nonetheless ITN would not have allowed him out on them if they had not thought he could do them. By now Kim's sights were set so high he did not realise how much of an achievement this was. The people at ITN had not expected him ever to be able to report a piece alone. Further proof of ITN's growing faith in him was when he was put back on the roster in July. Up until then he had been working four days a week always starting at ten in the morning, so if he was sent out it was planned, and he was never put in a position where he might be the only person on duty if a big story broke. Going back on the roster meant the beginning of being treated more like an ordinary reporter.

All this time Kim's father's health was deteriorating. I had not seen him since the previous summer but it was becoming apparent he was not likely to survive the coming winter. Kim had been down to Bristol quite often, and when in mid-July his father was admitted to hospital with stomach pains Kim went down again. He returned full of good cheer saying he and his father were getting on better than ever, and as the hospital could find nothing wrong with his father he was being sent home. He was not a man to make a fuss about nothing, so Kim constantly telephoned to make sure everything was all right. On the Monday after his visit his mother told him his father was too ill to speak to him, but should be better by the next time he called.

We were going out to dinner that night and as we drove there, for the first time I brought up the possibility of his father's death. I was worried about whether Kim would be able to deal with it. I said if there was another bad winter I did not think his father would live through it, he had been extremely ill during two of the last four winters, pulling himself through on willpower alone. This strength of character had not weakened but his body had taken the toll and I felt he could not survive another bout of bronchitis. The conversation upset Kim but it helped prepare him for his father's death.

The next day Little Sue, Kim's sister-in-law, rang to say his father was dead. The drugs he had been given to treat his stomach condition had proved too much and he had had a heart attack.

Kim put the phone down in tears, turned to me and in a few simple words poignantly expressed his sense of total loss: "I will never see him again."

He became worried that he had never told his father he loved him. I could honestly assure him that his father had never doubted Kim's love. He then became upset that his father would not see our baby. Far more important was that his father had lived to see Kim get better; that must have given him more pleasure than any number of Kim's children.

We went down to Bristol and stayed until after the funeral. Constantly at the back of my mind was the dread of going into labour with the strain of the occasion and the heat of those late July days.

On 6 August, thirteen days after Kim's father died, our son Pascoe Vicente Sabido was born. It was only a four-hour labour and I diligently did my breathing as I had been taught, but the last forty-five minutes were agony. The instant relief when I had finally pushed him out made me think the miracle of childbirth everybody talks about has nothing to do with the arrival of a new living thing in the world but is the sudden removal of all the pain. When the slimy little thing was handed to me I was not overcome by his beauty and said: "Oh, look. It's E.T." The nurses all assured me he was beautiful, but I was not fooled: with his large eyes, wide forehead and funny little expression he looked just like the little alien from the film. His lack of looks did not make me love him any the less. I felt immediately protectively maternal, believing that if I did not look after this funny little thing no one else would.

I had desperately wanted a girl, so my immediate reaction on being told the sex was: "All that effort just to get a boy out." The disappointment disappeared in seconds and has never returned.

We had agreed that if it was a boy it would be a Sabido (and if a girl MccGwire), but had reached an impasse over boys' names. Knowing I would be granted anything in the minutes immediately after labour I told Kim I wanted him to be called Pascoe after the man Duncan shared a house with. He had died of a heart attack while I was pregnant. I had spent many nights sitting round the kitchen giggling with Pascoe and Duncan and I wanted to remember him in some way.

Vicente was after Kim's father.

Kim was present at the birth and was so overwhelmed by it all that he was on another plane for days. When I had been taken up to the maternity ward Kim left the room to go to the loo just a few yards down the corridor. While he was out Duncan arrived and we talked for a while, then I began to wonder where Kim was. Twenty minutes later he turned up, having walked through most of the hospital. He had kept on forgetting where he was going and what he was doing and walked on and on. I was glad he had Duncan to look after him that night because he was obviously incapable of even getting himself home.

The months after Pascoe's birth proved I was right in thinking the baby would be a means of keeping us together. Without him we might not have survived. Of course I was exhausted by his constant demands; he put on weight at such a rate that while he was breastfeeding I sometimes wondered if I only ate to convert the food to milk to put into his stomach. But my focus was turned inwards to making a home for the three of us, which meant I constantly ministered to Kim's and the baby's needs.

Kim was starting on his most difficult time, the final steps on the ladder to 'normality': getting accepted as a reporter at ITN. He was constantly assigned to stories that did not make the bulletin. Night after night he would come home despondent and I would try to cheer him up, always pointing out how much progress he had made. I knew he was never going to achieve anything by feeling sorry for himself. If he was going to get back he had to fight for it. I understood how difficult it was for him but he had to keep his head up, grit his teeth and show everybody he was good enough to do it. It was going to be long and hard but it was the only way.

Pascoe gave Kim an outside interest, although not enough to make up for the constant humiliation he was feeling at work. I told him that he would look back on Pascoe's first couple of years and be grateful that he had taken so long to get back into the swing of things; they had developed a special relationship only possible with time and effort. Soon enough Kim would regain his place at ITN and be an absentee father. Already I never had any idea when he would be home from work. If he was given a story that was used he would not return until after ten, which happened about once a week, for all his despondency.

Around this time Kim showed me a letter he had written replying to someone congratulating him on being back at work, and in it he said it was Pascoe who kept him going when he found life unbearable. I think the fact that I was no longer a reporter also helped. If I had been working I would have been concerned with problems of my own and would have added to Kim's frustration because I would have been doing the sort of work that he wanted to do, and I would not have had the strength and patience for the support he needed. I wondered how many ordinary marriages required this constant ego massaging and encouragement and decided this was why men were such high achievers.

In early October we returned to Rivermead to see Barbara Wilson for a final assessment of Kim. When she rang to arrange the appointment she said she knew he had done pieces on television, obviously there had been a great deal of progress.

She was very kind and told both of us there was nothing she liked more than being proved wrong, and it was good that Kim was so much better. She said that when I took Kim out of Rivermead she thought I was putting too much pressure on him and he would crack under the strain; she had been very worried about it, but was pleased it had all worked out well. She gave Kim those terrible assessment tests again, and he did not get them right, so there were obviously still some problems.

We had lunch with her and discussed the other people in Kim's group. There had been about twenty of them and they had been divided into three groups when they left: those expected to get better, those expected to deteriorate and the ones who would stay the same. Kim had been rated in the last group: he would probably learn to cope with his problems better but there would be no actual improvement. Out of the twenty he was the only one who had managed to return to work. I felt sick at the wasted potential. If Kim could get back to his tough, demanding job, what had happened to the others after they left ?

A few months later I returned to Rivermead alone to ask Barbara why Kim had made it and the others had not. She said there were a variety of reasons. From what Kim had told her during that October visit it was apparent that he was using most of the memory aid techniques she had taught him, so he was making the best use of the memory he had. The crucial factor in Kim's case was the support he had, not just from me but also from ITN. Undoubtedly ITN had played a key role in his recovery because they had both looked after him and stretched him. Few employers would contemplate the kind of help ITN had given. Some did keep people's jobs open, but many did not. With high unemployment those who lost their jobs stood little chance of getting another, and with that goal removed they had little spur to recovery.

I rate Barbara Wilson extremely highly. She taught Kim a great deal and without the therapy he received at Rivermead he would not have been able to deal with *City Limits*, let alone ITN, and in spite of my deciding I knew better than she did, she has always been kind to the two of us. However, I do have two major areas of disagreement with her.

She believes that once the memory is damaged it cannot improve, one can only find ways round the difficulty. Over the years I have watched Kim's memory improve as he has been able to operate more and more like he used to, without relying on aids.

She also believes one should never raise anybody's expectations because they might be disappointed. She is in a difficult position because her patients' relatives can always say to her "but you said he would get better and he hasn't". However, I know that without my apparently unachievable expectations Kim would not have got better. If I had not always believed in him and forced him to try he just would have stayed hopelessly absentminded, unable to hold down a job. If I had believed Barbara I would have given up and so would he – he would never have made it. I believe in the power of hope.

For Kim's thirtieth birthday in December I planned a surprise party and it was a great success. He had no idea of what was awaiting him when he walked into our house at eight o'clock that evening to be greeted by about one hundred people singing Happy Birthday. He was wonderful, entering into the fun immediately and loving all the attention. My sister had bought him a funny hat with large felt flowers sticking out of it. He put it on and proceeded to get gloriously drunk. He went around in a daze for ages afterwards, overcome by how many people had turned up; he kept on saying he did not realise how many friends he had. It showed his sad lack of confidence.

In January I started working again. Pascoe was five months old and I was finding undiluted motherhood unsatisfying and needed to get my teeth into something more intellectually demanding. I decided not to go back to TV AM as the irregular hours would have meant I rarely saw Pascoe and I would have been torn between him and wanting to do my work properly. I became a freelance journalist doing both television and writing. Kim had improved immeasurably and although his close friends and family noticed he was not quite as he used to be, to anyone meeting him for the first time there appeared to be no problems. He easily managed his own life, there were no difficulties when I went away and, unlike most fathers, he was not daunted by looking after Pascoe alone when I was working at the weekend.

His sense of direction had not returned, but I just drew him maps of anywhere he was going to. He still had large memory gaps in the decade before the accident, which were slowly being filled, although occasionally he would muddle the chronology of events in his past. I felt there would be little further improvement until he had proved to himself that he could match up to ITN's standards.

The next few months were fairly awful as Kim went on slowly improving and fighting to get back at ITN. What made it so difficult for him was that he was worried that if he did get put on a good story he would mess it up, so he was not even sure he wanted to be given a chance to prove himself. There was nothing I could do except give him encouragement. Until he had conquered ITN nothing had any worth: he was always going to blame the accident for leaving a permanent scar on his life. It was no good telling him that to many people he had already achieved the impossible by just getting regular stories on the television. To people watching the news he was a success, but he measured himself against his colleagues and found himself wanting.

I was finding being Kim's emotional crutch exhausting, working as well as looking after Pascoe was enough of a strain without it. I clung on grimly, knowing eventually it would change.

The turning point was Stonehenge. One Saturday in May he was working a normal day shift. We had been invited to a barbecue that evening by Sue Inglish, so I rang him after the five o'clock news to ask what time he would be home. The news desk told me he was at Stonehenge and they did not know when he would return. He was still there at eight so I went without him, presuming he was doing a light piece on tourists or hippies.

Later that night Kim called me to tell me what had happened, still in shock from what he had seen. There had been quiet rumblings for some time over an argument about whether Stonehenge could be used to celebrate the summer solstice. This year the owners of Stonehenge, the National Trust, had obtained an injunction to keep people away, but many had declared their intention to break the injunction because they felt the National Trust had no right to ban people from such a sacred and symbolic site. A group calling themselves the Peace Convoy, who had been travelling around Wiltshire and the adjoining counties for a number of years, were continually harassed by the police. Various articles about them had appeared in the popular press painting them as dangerous desperadoes. When Nick Davies had been at the *Guardian* he had spent some time with them and was shocked to find the stories were exaggerations and fantasies. They were just ordinary people who had chosen to live an alternative life, and were bemused by the loathing they aroused.

That Saturday afternoon the Peace Convoy was slowly trundling towards Stonehenge, and the police decided it was time for a showdown.

Kim had been sent on the story very late, when the first reports of trouble arrived at ITN. By the time he arrived there was chaos. The travellers had gone into a field and were surrounded by police, who appeared to have gone berserk. Egged on by colleagues circling above in helicopters they hit out at anything in sight: vans, windows, people's heads – all came under their truncheons. Kim told me about the people he saw staggering out of their vans covered in blood, cowering from the police as they were hit. Women were desperately trying to shield their children from the blows, a baby was lying in a cot covered in broken glass from a window that had been smashed above him. Kim had never seen anything like it. This unprovoked brutality was far worse than the Falklands.

The only other journalist who witnessed it was Nick Davies, all the others had stayed behind the police lines, relying on them for their information, which was rather different from the eye-witness accounts. Kim's piece on television combined with Nick's lead article in the *Observer* the next day ensured the rest of the country knew the truth about what had happened.

When Kim came home he had a stature and confidence I had not seen before. Finally he knew he could do it. There were still months of ups and downs ahead, but he had started the final ascent up the ITN ladder. I felt that because he had gone back too early and people at ITN had seen him so vulnerable and unsure of himself they had taken longer to trust him.

It finally proved we were right to aim high. Many times over the previous eighteen months I had wondered if I was wise to push so hard. It would have been so much easier for both of us if Kim had been content to be just a minion at ITN. But in general after a head injury I am sure it is important to aim high in order to achieve maximum potential. It is equally important constantly to remind oneself this is not a mentally handicapped person and must not be treated like one. Relatively few people have as far to go as Kim had. However disparaging one might be about the ability needed to be a journalist, he was at the top of an aggressive, competitive and highly pressurised business.

As he conquered work the equilibrium of our relationship began slowly to improve. Trying to nurture it into an independent meeting of minds would be our next task. Having come this far together did not mean we would not part, for I was worried about the problem of over exposure. For months we had had a nurse-patient relationship, with me caring for Kim and supporting him while he used me as an emotional crutch. It would be difficult for us to return to looking at each other through the eyes of lovers. For our relationship to work this had to happen. It was our final hurdle and one we would have to get over together. There were times when I wondered if we could ever recapture the magic we had had.

When I was talking about this book to Tom Rayner, Kim's friend whom he met after the TV Eye film and who had had a head injury himself, I told him that I wanted to provide encouragement to all the people like me who found themselves suddenly having to deal with a brain-damaged person. He said he realised it was tough for those who had to deal with the patients, but what I had to bear in mind was that however awful it was for me it was a hundred times worse for Kim, who had been trapped in his shell. Unlike me, he had had no choice.

It is something I have always remembered.